Contents

About the author

Theresa Cheung is the author of numerous health and popular psychology books, including *The Glycaemic Factor: How to Balance Your Blood Sugar* and *How to Boost Your Immune System*. She also co-authored the best-selling *PCOS Diet Book* and has contributed features to *Here's Health, NHS Mother and Baby, You Are What You Eat, Red* and *Prima* magazines.

CAR

Overcoming Common Problems

The IBS Healing Plan

THERESA CHEUNG

sheldon**PRESS**

First published in Great Britain in 2007

Sheldon Press
36 Causton Street
London SW1P 4ST

British Library Cataloguing-in-Publication Data
A catalogue record for this book is available from the British Library

ISBN 978–1–84709–013–3

1 3 5 7 9 10 8 6 4 2

Typeset by Fakenham Photosetting Ltd, Fakenham, Norfolk
Printed in Great Britain. by Ashford Colour Press

Produced on paper from sustainable forests

Introduction: Problems 'down there'

As far as health problems go, irritable bowel is way down the bottom of the list (no pun intended!) People don't have a problem openly discussing diabetes, hypertension and even PMS, but mention the bowels and people get ill at ease.

It's not hard to understand why: how on earth to do you slip in to normal conversation, 'I had terrible diarrhoea last week and it got so bad I pooped myself in my car because I couldn't find a toilet in time.' What on earth would you expect anyone to say in response to that anyway? Or, try telling your colleagues why it would not be a good idea to have you present to some important clients: 'I'd like to, really I would, but the chances are I'll be constipated for days beforehand and then about five minutes before the meeting starts my colon will spasm and I'll have to spend the next few hours apologizing every ten minutes because I've got the runs and need to rush to the bathroom.' It's also not hard to understand why irritable bowel gets very little attention from the press and media. What reporter wants someone talking about his or her uncontrollable bowel movements on air? And just how would you go about persuading a celebrity to be the face of an awareness campaign – or attracting corporate sponsors to fund awareness and research?

Although people don't like to talk about it much, there is no escaping the fact that Irritable Bowel Syndrome (IBS) is a widespread condition that affects about one in five Europeans and Americans. These are pretty serious statistics for an ailment described as just being 'irritable'. Yet in a society where bowel dysfunction is not considered a topic of polite conversation, it can be difficult to find help for IBS. In fact, according to the International Foundation for Functional Gastrointestinal Disorders (IFFGD), most of those with IBS may not be getting the medical attention they need. If you think you may be one of these people, then it's time to read this book, trust your gut, and get to grips with your discomfort using *The IBS Healing Plan*.

The symptoms of IBS differ from person to person, and can involve any number or combination of the following: intestinal spasm, constipation, diarrhoea, haemorrhoids or anal fissures (small tears in the anus caused by excessive straining or hard stools or frequent bowel movements). Depending on how severe and frequent symptoms are, IBS can either be a minor irritation or something that destroys the quality of your life. Sadly, medical treatments for IBS don't always help, and some have side effects that are even worse than the symptoms themselves. For example, some anti diarrhoea medications can make some people with IBS bloat like a beach ball and expel loud, noisy wind all the time, to the extent that even the diarrhoea was preferable. The good news is that there are a number of natural therapies for IBS that can be quite effective; you'll find them all clearly explained in this book.

Many people who have IBS try to overlook it, but it can't and shouldn't be ignored for long. *The IBS Healing Plan* confirms that IBS is real and shows you the many ways you can successfully deal with your symptoms, working with or without the help of your doctor. Because there is no wonder drug for IBS, those who have the condition often try all sorts of therapies for relief. This book sorts through all the available remedies, and outlines only the best and most effective ones. In short, it presents a practical, holistic approach to the condition that will help you, or a loved one if you are reading this book for someone else, leave the wind, pain and strain and other problems 'down there' behind – for good.

1
What is IBS?

Jack, 47
I was diagnosed with IBS about two years ago. Like most of us I have had both good days, bad days and truly foul days.

About three months ago I had a lunch meeting with a client from out of town. Things felt good business-wise and IBS-wise and after the lunch I headed back to my car to drive to my office. I felt the familiar IBS discomfort, but it was mild and, knowing that my office was only a ten-minute drive away, I thought it would be fine. It wasn't.

After five minutes in the car the traffic came to an unexpected halt. I was at a standstill for about ten minutes and I started to wish I had used the loo at the restaurant. I put the radio on and heard that there had been an accident close by and there would be delays of up to 30 minutes. I knew I didn't have 30 minutes.

I decided to drive up the wrong side of the road so that I could take a right turn that would take me to another street which led to my office. What I didn't know was that three cars behind me there was a police motorbike, and the next thing I knew was that there were red flashing lights in my rear view mirror. I pulled over and, squirming with embarrassment, told the policewoman that I wouldn't normally break the law like that but I have IBS and I *have* to find a loo. Sadly, she was not sympathetic and wrote out a ticket for an illegal turn. By the time she had handed it to me, it was too late. My pants were full and I had stained the car seat. I had no choice but to call the office and say I needed the rest of the day off.

Tracey, 29
I became nervous about my bowel symptoms when a friend of mine was diagnosed with colon cancer. I don't know what symptoms she was having, but it got me very concerned. I went to my doctor, and he did a thorough examination and asked me a lot of questions. He said that my symptoms were very similar to those of people who have irritable bowel syndrome. I asked him how he could be sure without doing any tests. He said that he couldn't be absolutely sure, but that he was confident that I didn't have anything more serious. I told him that I really

was concerned, and that I would feel better if we did some tests. So I am doing some home treatment and going in next week for some tests. Even if they don't show anything, I know that I will rest easier.

Linda, 33

My daughter and I were renting a holiday cottage by the beach, which had only one bathroom. She was in the bathroom when I had to go. I had to use the cats' litter tray as I had forgotten to bring along my porta-potty.

While on holiday I made so many trips to the bathroom that my daughter thought I had taken up residence there. At one point while in the bathroom I started to think about potty as an Olympic event, with styles of rolling the toilet paper and styles of wiping and toilet dismount. Seriously, though, IBS has ruined my holiday and ruins most of my outings when I have to tear through places to get to the toilet.

Mark, 18

I'm 18 in a few months' time, and since having IBS I've seen myself deteriorate very fast. The first time I got constipated it was so bad I had to go to the hospital to have suppositories put up me. It was so embarrassing and really painful. It felt like I had years full of waste inside of me that needed to come out but wouldn't. I was given strong painkillers and anti-sickness tablets to help with me being sick every time I strained on the toilet.

When I went home, I did manage to go to the toilet, but I wasn't going much and it was painful. I always left the toilet weaker and more fragile than when I went in. Then my second attack came, worse than my first. I hadn't been able to go for a week and the cramping was excruciating. I had no energy to go back to the hospital again. I had no choice either. Off I went and had the same treatment as before. I had an interview in a few weeks' time for a job I really wanted, but how could I do a job when I get sudden attacks of IBS?

I'm scared of taking drugs. In fact, I'm scared of everything, even going out of the house. I don't know how to deal with it any more, it's embarrassing to me. And I have no idea why this has happened to me, why don't any of my friends who eat junk all day long have this problem?

If these IBS (irritable bowel syndrome) stories from Jack, Mark, Linda and Tracey strike a cord with you, the chances are you have IBS or know someone who does. But what exactly is IBS?

One of the most important weapons in your battle against IBS – also called spastic colon and mucous colitis – is information. You need to know the enemy. Fortunately, over the past few years a great deal of new information regarding the brain–gut interaction that results in IBS has evolved, and more discoveries are being made all the time.

First of all, it helps to realize that you are not alone. IBS is estimated to affect 15–20 per cent of people, and half of them have never even seen a doctor for their symptoms. Despite this, IBS is still the most frequently seen condition by gastroenterologists, and is one of the top ten diagnoses among all US and UK doctors. It is also, incredibly, the second leading cause of worker absenteeism (behind only the common cold). These are pretty amazing statistics for a condition that some people have never even heard of or regard as a very minor ailment.

Interestingly, because IBS is a 'functional' condition, you can't actually be tested for it. Rather, it is determined by a diagnosis of exclusion. This is because there aren't actually any structural, inflammatory, biochemical or infectious abnormalities present in IBS. In other words, when those with IBS are examined by doctors, there is no physical problem to be found. So, are you just imagining your symptoms? No – you absolutely are not! A functional disorder simply means that the problem is an altered physiological function (that is, the way your body works), rather than something that has an identifiable origin behind it. In other words, while an IBS attack and its resulting symptoms are clearly visible as physical manifestations, the underlying cause behind these symptoms is not. Put another way, the root of the problem in those with IBS cannot yet be identified by yielding a positive result from any existing medical tests. So what then, precisely, is wrong with the way your body works if you have IBS?

IBS is indisputably a physical and mental problem. Simply put, the brain–gut interaction of people with IBS influences their bowel pain perception and motility. The processing of pain information within the central nervous system varies between those free of IBS and those who have the condition, with the result that the latter group can experience even normal gastrointestinal (GI) contractions as painful. The interactions between the brains, central nervous systems and GI systems of those with IBS are just not functioning properly. They have colons that react to stimuli that do not affect normal colons, and their reactions are much more severe. The end result is heightened pain sensitivity and abnormal gut motility, in the form of irregular or increased GI muscle contractions. It is this gut overreaction and altered pain perceptions that cause the lower abdominal cramping, pain, wind and accompanying diarrhoea and/or constipation that characterize IBS.

To fully understand IBS, it's also important to recognize what it is *not*. IBS is not a form of bowel cancer or an inflammatory disease such as Crohn's or coeliac disease (though it can be secondary to these), nor a condition that leads to other life-threatening illnesses. While it is still a complex functional disorder, IBS merely relates to a set of symptoms that fail to indicate disease in diagnostic tests, and these symptoms include cramping, bloating, wind, diarrhoea and constipation, vomiting, mucus in the stools, and a full sensation after even a small meal.

To sum up, although medical researchers aren't exactly sure what IBS is, it equates to bowel discomfort and irritation that can either send you running to the loo faster than the speed of light or desperately reaching for a laxative. Like an unannounced visitor who drops in when you're just about to go out, or the annoying caller who won't let you off the phone, IBS comes calling whenever and wherever it likes.

Diagnosing irritable bowel syndrome

According to the IFFGD (International Foundation for Functional Gastrointestinal Disorders), clinical IBS is characterized by at least 12 weeks out of a 12-month period of abdominal pain or discomfort, recurrent diarrhoea and/or constipation (conditions that should always prompt a visit to the doctor to rule out other causes).

As we have seen, IBS is diagnosed by its symptoms, not by a particular medical test. This is because, as mentioned above, an irritable bowel is a normal, healthy bowel that for some reason does not co-ordinate its functions properly. Distressing as a diagnosis of IBS is, never forget that it does not lead to bowel cancer or other serious bowel disorders such as colitis, Crohn's disease and others.

Symptoms of IBS

The symptoms of IBS depend on which parts of the gut are involved. Some people may experience problems in only one part of the gut, others in several. Symptoms are unpredictable and can also vary over time. For example, for several months, weeks or days you may suffer from bouts of diarrhoea, and then for several months, weeks or days you may suffer from constipation. Listed below are typical symptoms and the parts of the digestive system involved.

Symptoms relating to the oesophagus

- A sensation like a golf ball in the throat between meals which does not interfere with swallowing.
- Heartburn – a burning pain that is often felt behind the breastbone.
- Painful swallowing, but without the hold-up of food.

Symptoms relating to the stomach

- Non-ulcer dyspepsia (symptoms suggestive of a stomach or duodenal ulcer, but that has not been confirmed on investigation).
- Feeling full after small meals. This may reach the stage of not being able to finish a meal.
- Abdominal bloating after meals.

Symptoms relating to the small bowel

- Increased gurgling noises that may be loud enough to cause social embarrassment.
- Abdominal bloating that may be so severe that women describe themselves as looking pregnant.
- Generalized abdominal tenderness associated with bloating.
- Abdominal bloating of both types that usually subsides overnight and returns the following day.

Symptoms relating to the large bowel

- Abdominal bloating of both types (see above list) which usually subsides overnight and returns the following day.
- Right-sided abdominal pain, either low or tucked up under the right-hand ribs. This does not always get better on opening the bowels.
- Pain tucked up under the left-hand ribs. When the pain is bad, it may enter the left armpit.
- Variable and erratic bowel habits alternating from constipation to diarrhoea.
- Increased gastro-colic reflex. This is an awakening of the reflex where food in the stomach stimulates colonic activity, resulting in the need to open the bowels.
- Severe, short stabbing pains in the rectum, called proctalgia fugax.

Other symptoms associated with IBS

- Headaches.
- In women, left-sided abdominal pain during sex.
- Passing urine more frequently.
- Fatigue and tiredness.

- Mucus in stools
- Sleep disturbance.
- Loss of appetite.
- Nausea.
- Depressive symptoms in about a third of those with IBS.
- Anxiety and stress-related symptoms, which may interact with gut symptoms.

Doctors look for a specific pattern of symptoms when making a diagnosis, and if you have at least three of the six most common symptoms – abdominal pain, infrequency of bowel movements with bouts of diarrhoea and/or constipation, mucus in the stools, a sensation of incomplete emptying of the rectum after going to the bathroom, and a bloated or distended feeling in the abdomen – then you meet the criteria for a diagnosis of IBS.

Symptoms that should not be ascribed to IBS

Because IBS can mimic so many other intestinal disorders, it's important to identify those symptoms that are not connected to IBS but can easily be confused with IBS. If any of the following occur, you should see your doctor immediately:

- Difficulty in swallowing and when food gets stuck.
- Indigestion-type pain that wakes you up during the night.
- Abdominal bloating that does not get better overnight.
- Significant and unexplained weight loss.
- Bleeding from the back passage.
- Chronic, painless diarrhoea.

This list is not comprehensive. If you are experiencing other symptoms, you should seek further advice.

(*Note*: Although IBS can be a distressing condition and never causes bowel cancer or bowel damage, first-time symptoms of what seem to be IBS in a person, especially those over the age of 40, should in general be assessed by a doctor.)

2

What causes IBS?

Sally, 26
I get really frustrated when doctors minimize the impact that IBS has made on my life. Just because my doctor can't find anything on the lab tests and has no idea what is causing my problems, he tells me it's not worth worrying about. That's easy for him to say. IBS has ruined my social life. I can't even enjoy dinner with my boyfriend without worrying about ending up like a hot-air balloon at the end of the night.

Interestingly, the origins of IBS may really be in our brains, and not in our bowels. Given that for many years people with IBS were told dismissively that their problem was 'all in their heads', it's ironic that, in the end, this may be factually correct. The underlying problem might well be in your brain, but this does *not* mean it is in your imagination.

Although research is ongoing, no one really knows yet exactly why some people develop IBS and others don't. A great deal of research has been devoted to discovering the causes, especially the gut and brain interaction, but while we have learned a lot, crucial questions remain unanswered.

For many years, researchers thought that IBS was caused by poorly co-ordinated muscular contractions in the gut, but studies have shown that although people with IBS do sometimes have this problem, it does not always occur. As a result, doctors and medical researchers have had to look elsewhere for other possible causes. Here's a round-up of the latest research conclusions:

Is IBS inherited?

Often IBS seems to 'run in the family', thus raising the possibility that IBS is an inherited condition. When confronted with such questions of 'nature versus nurture', investigators often study identical twins raised apart; however, these studies are quite difficult, as the number of such twins available for study is obviously limited. Talley and his colleagues in Australia reported on the GI symptoms experienced by 437 pairs of twins with abdominal pain, and found that irritable bowel symptoms occurred in both twins to a greater degree than would be expected by chance alone, but was far from 100 per cent. Thus, they concluded that although genetics may in part explain the occurrence of IBS, other environmental factors must be involved.

IBS and food intolerance

Studies show that between 33 per cent and 66 per cent of those with IBS report having one or more food intolerances. The most common culprits are dairy products (40–44 per cent) and grains (40–60 per cent). The fact that some but not all of those with IBS report food intolerances suggests that it is not the primary cause. (If you think certain foods may be causing or triggering symptoms, be sure to read the dietary advice in Chapter 4: Healing IBS with diet.)

Is there a neurochemical imbalance in IBS?

Interaction or communication between the brain and the gut occurs via nerves that send neurotransmitter signals. An imbalance between two of these neurotransmitters, serotonin and norepinephrine, are implicated in IBS. Constipation may result when levels of norepinephrine increase, causing a reduction in serotonin levels and the inhibition of another neurotransmitter called acetylcholine. Conversely, diarrhoea can occur when increased serotonin inhibits norepinephrine and causes levels of acetylcholine to increase. If this all sounds a bit technical, in short it means, for those with IBS, that such an imbalance in the nervous system can lead to the fluctuating bowel symptoms of constipation and diarrhoea. Research on nerve function is spearheading IBS research at the present time, and there is evidence to suggest that there may well be differences in the brains of people with IBS and in the way they experience bowel movements.

IBS and analgesics

The use of acetaminophen, a common pain-relieving medication, is associated with diarrhoea-predominant IBS. Its action may be due to an imbalance in the neurotransmitter serotonin. Since acetaminophen can cause elevated levels of the serotonin by-product 5-HIAA in the urine, it is possible that acetaminophen somehow interferes with serotonin metabolism. Plasma serotonin levels have indeed been shown to be elevated after eating in those with diarrhoea-predominant IBS. Clinically, a drug that blocks the 5-HT3 serotonin receptor (5-HT3 receptor antagonist) is effective for women with diarrhoea-predominant IBS.

The role of reproductive hormones

IBS occurs more than twice as frequently in women than in men and tends to follow a cyclical pattern, with aggravation during the post-ovulatry (progesterone-dominant) and premenstrual phases of the menstrual cycle. Progesterone is known to delay gastric emptying and cause constipation. Constipation with straining and the frequent passage of hard stools is a more prevalent IBS manifestation in women, especially during the post-ovulatory or PMS phase, which is about 14 days before a period. At the end of the post-ovulatory phase, the sudden withdrawal of progesterone that occurs with the start of the premenstrual phase may trigger increased bowel activity. Women frequently report loose stools and diarrhoea before or with the onset of menstruation. In contrast to progesterone, oestrogen has not been associated with exacerbations of IBS symptoms.

In one study, high levels of the reproductive hormone luteinizing hormone (LH) were found in women with IBS. Drugs that decreased LH levels, and consequently suppressed ovarian production of oestrogen and progesterone, resulted in significantly improved IBS symptoms. LH is a reproductive hormone responsible for the production of testosterone in males and oestrogen and progesterone in women. In men, the opposite result was found: low LH and low testosterone (male hormone) tended to be associated with IBS symptoms. High LH therefore appears to cause exacerbations in women by stimulating progesterone and oestrogen, yet it appears to have a protective effect in men.

Along with progesterone levels in women, prostaglandins E2 and F2 alpha also increase in the premenstrual phase. Since they are powerful stimulants of bowel contractions, it is possible that women with IBS may have an exaggerated response to these prostaglandins. (If you are a woman and suffer from increased bloating and constipation the week before your period, and looser bowel movements during your period, the advice in Chapter 9 about cyclical symptoms of IBS and PMS will prove helpful.)

Mood and IBS

Anxiety, hostile feelings, sadness, depression and sleep disturbance are associated with IBS. Adverse life events such as a family death, marital stress, financial difficulties, and especially physical and sexual abuse, have also been reported more frequently in people with IBS than in the general population. However, it is possible that people with IBS with this social or psychological background may be more likely to seek medical treatment or participate in research studies.

The impact of stress on bowel motility and pain was explored in one study by administering corticotrophin-releasing factor (CRF), a hormone released in the body during stress. CRF increases motility of the descending colon and can induce abdominal pain. The researchers found that those with IBS had greater colonic motility and more abdominal pain after receiving CRF than controls.

Bacterial overgrowth in the small intestine

An overgrowth of bacteria in the small intestine, an area that is normally relatively free of bacteria, is being recognized as important in the development of IBS. When these bacteria are present in the small intestine, excessive wind, bloating, abdominal distension and pain, and altered gut motility, can result.

Causes of small-intestine bacterial overgrowth include decreased gastric acid secretion (possibly due to natural ageing, stomach ulcers and colonization by *Helicobacter pylori* bacteria), decreased bile flow, or decreased pancreatic enzymes with poor absorption of carbohydrates, fats and proteins. The resulting undigested and unabsorbed carbohydrates in the small intestine and colon cause excess fermentation and encourage growth of unwanted bacterial species. An abundance of gas is produced, as well as short-chain organic acids such as lactic acid, which can damage the mucous lining of the intestines and further contribute to poor absorption of carbohydrates. In addition, putrefaction of proteins in the small intestine produces substances called vasoactive amines that can affect intestinal muscles.

There is mounting evidence that for some people with IBS the condition is precipitated by some type of grievous insult to the gut – dysentery, food poisoning, intestinal flu, abdominal surgery, even pregnancy. The theory goes that even after full physical recovery from these traumatic events, the nerves within the gut retain a 'memory' of the insult and remain hyper-sensitive to further stimulation, as well as prone to excess bacteria and subsequent over-reaction.

Gut dysbiosis

Some experts believe that IBS is associated with a condition known as gut dysbiosis, sometimes called leaky gut syndrome. We all have bacteria in our guts and it is vital for good digestion and the health of the intestines. Unfortunately, the body can often become infested with bad bacteria and when this happens levels of good bacteria are lowered and digestion is compromised. When there is an overgrowth of bad versus good bacteria in your gut, dysbiosis occurs.

Even though research has not yet confirmed a firm link between gut dysbiosis and IBS, to have this condition is bad news for a number of reasons:

- With digestion compromised, gut dysbiosis can trigger stomach upsets, bloating, constipation and diarrhoea – all symptoms of IBS.
- It produces toxins that can damage the intestinal walls, and prevent good bacteria from producing their healthy organic acids which support colon health.
- To function effectively, your immune system needs nutritional back-up, so when digestion is compromised, immunity is as well and so you become more susceptible to any other infections, viruses and diseases.
- Good bacteria aid food digestion and the production of vitamins and minerals, but gut dysbiosis limits the productivity of good diges-tion and causes nutritional deficiencies. If you are not getting the nutrients you need from your food, you'll feel unwell and tired.
- The bad bacteria and the toxins they create can make your gut hyper-permeable and more likely to allow unwanted particles into your bloodstream. This can cause your immune system to be on high alert all the time, as it does not recognize these foreign particles and the result is food allergies, mysterious aches and pains, inflam-mation, fatigue, dizziness, foggy mind and poor concentration.

Stress is believed to be a trigger for gut dysbiosis. Experts argue that we have a second more primitive 'brain' located in the stomach area; this is because there is a large concentration of nerves in the area of the stomach. We all have butterflies in our stomachs when we feel anxious, frightened or stressed. Your stomach and intestines are very sensitive to stress, and when you feel stressed, digestion shuts down to help the body focus on preparing the flight and fight response. This means that food is only partially digested, leading to gut dysbiosis and nutrient deficiency. If stress is long term, in time the body gradually becomes less able to produce stomach acid and digestive enzymes because it is now deficient in vitamins and minerals required for these enzymes, and a vicious circle occurs. Another trigger for gut dysbiosis is thought to be a poor diet high in sugar, refined carbohydrates and processed food because it deprives the body of nutrients, compromises digestion, limits the productivity of good bacteria and feeds bad bacteria in the gut. Unfortunately, the standard Western diet is high in refined carbohydrates, sugar and low in fibre, protein and fresh uncooked fruit and vegetables – a recipe for leaky gut and, some might say, IBS symptoms.

Your early warning sign

The possible causes outlined above offer fascinating insights into why some people get IBS and some don't, but none of them fully explains the condition, and there are still those who are exceptions to every theory and who are still patiently waiting for an explanation. Despite this, the work of researchers is invaluable as it can lead to better ways to understand and manage the condition. For example, new medications have been developed to relieve specific conditions, understanding that your gut may be prone to bacterial overgrowth may encourage you to find ways to maintain a healthy bowel lining with probiotic supplements, and recognizing that stress and poor diet may be a trigger can help you to avoid or find ways to manage stress and nutritional deficiency.

Right now the best approach to understanding IBS is to think of it as an early warning sign for you to step back and take a look at your diet and lifestyle. By learning your own triggers you can take control of your symptoms and lead an IBS-free life. Chapters 4 to 9 of this book will help you do just that, but before we launch into the IBS Healing Plan, let's first make sure that you, or someone you know if you are reading this book to help him or her, actually has IBS.

3

Do I have IBS?

Take some time to answer the questions below and read the accompanying information as your answers will help you identify whether or not you have IBS.

1 Do you have recurring bouts of abdominal pain?

Recurring bouts of abdominal pain for at least three months is the number one symptom of IBS. This pain is often located in the bottom part of the abdomen below the belly button, but it can be felt all over the abdomen. The pain tends to decrease after a bowel movement. Although pain is common with IBS and does not indicate serious disease, you should still check with your doctor if the pain has recently appeared or is very severe.

2 Are your bowel movements abnormal?

Many people have one or two, even three, bowel movements a day, typically in the morning, and this is considered perfectly normal. If you have more than three or four bowel movements a day and less than one bowel movement a day, your bowel movements are considered abnormal. Bear in mind that we all have days or times in our lives when bowel movements are irregular for a few days or even weeks due to a change in routine (your bowels love routine!), such as a holiday or change of job or house, or a stressful event (for example, a divorce), but once you settle into a routine again your bowel movements should return to normal. If they don't, IBS could be the problem.

3 Have your bowel movements changed?

Another common symptom of IBS is irregular bowel movement patterns interspersed with normal bowel function. For example, you could have irregular movements for one week out of every four.

4   Is there mucus in your stools?

Many people worry that the presence of mucus in their stools indicates serious bowel disease, but mucus without blood is a common finding in people with IBS. Mucus is a normal by-product of the bowel and serves as a lubricant. A symptom of IBS is more mucus than necessary, just as a runny nose is a symptom of a cold.

5   Do you suffer from bloating or abdominal swelling?

Yet another unpleasant and common symptom of IBS, bloating is usually worse after eating and in the evening. It often disappears or improves overnight.

6   After a bowel movement, do you experience a sensation of incomplete emptying of the rectum?

You may strain unnecessarily after a bowel movement to try and pass a stool. You have in fact completed your bowel movement, but the feeling of incomplete emptying is caused by the increased sensitivity of the gut. However, you should consult your doctor if you experience this persistently.

7   Do other non-bowel symptoms accompany your IBS?

You may experience any one of the following non-bowel symptoms alongside your IBS: heartburn, fatigue, urinary problems, migraines and painful intercourse.

If you answered yes to at least three of the questions above and have experienced these symptoms for more than three months, the chances are you have IBS. If you feel that your symptoms do not exactly fit with IBS, then it is vital that you see your doctor immediately.

Research studies have shown that the symptoms of IBS vary and may occur at any age. They most commonly start in the late teens or early adulthood and most people start to experience symptoms before they are 30. In fact, if you are over 40 and have IBS for the first time, you should see your doctor as it could be caused by a recent intestinal infection.

As we saw in Chapters 1 and 2, IBS occurs because for some reason the bowel is more sensitive than usual and there are problems with co-ordination of the bowel. IBS also seems to be more common in women than in men both in Europe and the USA. Curiously, in India more men report symptoms, although we don't know why this is.

Another distinguishing feature of IBS is that it does not always occur persistently and symptoms can, and do, come and go over time, often triggered by dietary changes and stress.

The chances are you may have looked into over-the-counter medications, such as laxatives, to relieve your symptoms, but the problem with long-term and frequent use of drugs is that they can actually make your symptoms worse because they aggravate your gut even more. No one drug can treat all the symptoms of IBS and, as the majority of people experience symptoms on and off throughout their lives, it would not be wise for these perfectly healthy individuals to take drugs for 30 or 40 years, especially when most drugs have potential side-effects. That's why it's best to avoid relying on drugs as much as possible and to use the natural healing techniques recommended in the chapters that follow.

Key statistics

1 Irritable bowel syndrome (IBS) is often confused with other conditions. It has been called by many names – colitis, mucous colitis, spastic colon, spastic bowel and functional bowel disease. Most of these terms are inaccurate. Colitis, for instance, means inflammation of the large intestine (the colon), while IBS doesn't cause inflammation.

2 IBS symptoms affect up to 20 per cent of the general population. It is the most common disorder diagnosed by gastroenterologists, and is among the most common health disorders in general.

3 Women are two to three times more likely than men to suffer from IBS. Moreover, they seem to have more symptoms during their periods, suggesting that reproductive hormones play a role.

4 IBS is a chronic condition – you might develop it in your late twenties and have it for years, even for the rest of your life. Fortunately, the symptoms may come and go. The late twenties are the typical age of onset.

5 IBS can be triggered by stress, and flare-ups of symptoms are associated with major stressful life events in the majority of those with the condition. Studies indicate that some psychological treatments, such as cognitive behavioural therapy, can alleviate abdominal pain and diarrhoea associated with the syndrome.

4

Healing IBS with diet

Research makes it clear that diet plays a direct role in gut function (something that is instinctively obvious to those with IBS) and symptoms are quite often triggered (not caused) by diet and dietary habits. Overeating, poor eating habits and eating certain foods can cause trouble. Some types of food that typically irritate the colon are:

- Foods high in fat.
- Spicy foods.
- Foods that contain caffeine such as coffee, tea, chocolate and soda.
- Alcohol.
- Avocados.
- Citrus fruits.
- Corn.
- Milk and diary products.
- Sugar.
- Wheat.

If you think that any of these foods are a literal pain in the colon for you, the solution is simple: stop eating them immediately and see if your symptoms improve after a week.

Jo, 30

I went to my doctor two years ago and was diagnosed with IBS. He told me to switch to a bland diet. I didn't want to take drugs, so he put the focus on healing with food. As he suggested, I ate stacks of fibre-rich food, but it didn't help at all. I read some IBS books and went on the internet to some IBS websites and decided to cut out all dairy products, animal protein, sugar and most fats. My symptoms got a little better, but I'd still have a few days every month when I was chained to the loo. A friend of mine – who has also got IBS – told me that chocolate might be making things worse for me. It was really tough for me to give up chocolate as I adore it and have a few bars every day, but within a few days of giving up chocolate my cramps disappeared. It's depressing for me to have had to give up something I adore, but there's no way I'd risk the pain and cramping again.

Start with healthy eating

If you've visited your doctor it's probable that she or he has already suggested a change in diet, typically an increase in fibre, in the hope that this will relieve discomfort and normalize your bowel movements. Healthy eating is the first step to easing the discomfort of IBS. The second step is to adjust your eating habits based on what we know about the eating-related causes of irritable bowel. Many people with IBS jump immediately to the second step and skip the first, but laying the foundation with a healthy diet is crucial because your body needs adequate nutrition to function optimally and help you to cope with stress.

There's so much advice out there in magazines, books and on the internet it can be hard to know what exactly a healthy diet is. The basic steps to good nutrition come from a diet that:

- Is balanced overall, with foods from all food groups, with lots of delicious fresh fruits, fresh vegetables, fresh wholegrains, and fat-free or low-fat milk and milk products.
- Is low in saturated fats, trans-fats and cholesterol and keeps total fat intake around 20 to 25 per cent of calories, with most fats coming from sources of polyunsaturated and monounsaturated fatty acids, such as fish, nuts, seeds and vegetable oils.
- Includes a variety of wholefoods, a good source of fibre; ideally around 50 per cent of total calories should be taken in the form of wholefoods, including grains along with lashings of fruit and vegetables. (Wholegrains may be a trigger food for some people with IBS, so refer to the advice below on soluble and insoluble fibre.)
- Includes a variety of fruits and vegetables. Eat at least five to seven servings of fruits and vegetables per day. They are an important source of vitamins, minerals, fibre and phytochemicals. Phytochemicals provide disease-protective effects to the body.
- Includes high-quality protein in the form of nuts, seeds, fish, lean meat and wholegrains; ideally around 20 per cent of our calories should come from protein.
- Has foods prepared with less sodium or salt because a high intake of sodium in the diet increases the risk of high blood pressure (aim for no more than about one teaspoonful of salt per day).
- Includes plenty of fluids, ideally in the form of water (six to eight glasses a day typically recommended) or juices.

The nutrients in food are fuel and you need that fuel to feel well, digest your food efficiently, function normally and cope with stress. Making sure your diet is healthy and that you have adequate nutrition from a balanced intake of carbohydrates, proteins and healthy fats, with at least six to eight glasses of water a day, is an essential foundation for good health, whether you have IBS or not.

Carbohydrates and IBS

When eaten, carbohydrates are broken down into glucose. We need glucose because it is the major fuel for the brain, muscles and immune system. Complex carbohydrates (i.e. unrefined foods, such as grains, fruit, vegetables, nuts and seeds) are by far the best way to get your carbohydrates, as they are packed with nutrients and great for your digestion and energy levels. Refined carbohydrates (i.e. processed foods, such as cakes, sweets, ready meals and white bread) flood the system with sugar as soon as they are eaten, providing a quick flash of energy followed by fatigue. In contrast, unrefined carbohydrates release their sugar slowly so that the blood sugar level stays in the normal range instead of going up and down rapidly. When blood sugar is low we crave sweets and become easily angry or anxious, but if it is steady we can concentrate better and don't have food cravings. Another benefit of unrefined carbohydrates is that they are high in fibre; this boosts digestion, removes toxins and encourages regular bowel movements.

Protein and IBS

Protein is the basic building block of all living cells. Proteins make up hormones, enzymes, antibodies and immune cells, and adequate protein intake is essential for your health and well-being. The constituents of protein are amino acids; there are eight that are vital to life and they can be found in lean meat, fish, low-fat dairy produce as well as beans, lentils nuts and seeds. Amino acids perform essential functions. Some control memory, sleep, mood, energy levels and how our digestive system functions. A poor diet can easily create an amino acid deficiency. Healthy forms of complete protein (i.e. they contain all eight essential amino acids) include quinoa, tofu, fish, lean chicken and combined pulses and grains.

Water and IBS

Water is the body's single most important nutrient. Almost all of the body's functions, including our immune system, rely on water. It carries nutrients to the cells; carries waste and toxins away from the cells and out of the body; maintains the body's temperature; and provides protection and cushioning for the joints and organs of the body as well as the skin. We lose water constantly through physiological processes such as sweating, elimination and breathing. This water needs to be replenished. The body does not keep a reserve of water as it does with other nutrients, so our need for water is continuous. Experts recommend that a healthy adult should drink around eight glasses of water per day. Sometimes we need more water because of accelerated loss of water due to heat, excessive sweating, diarrhoea, etc. Don't wait until you feel thirsty to drink water, as thirst is a sign of dehydration.

Avoid ice-cold foods and drinks on an empty stomach. Cold makes muscles contract, and your goal is to keep your stomach and the rest of your digestive system as calm as possible. And although you need to drink fresh water constantly throughout the day (not ice cold), you should limit the amount of water or other fluids you drink with your meals as this can inhibit digestion.

Healthy fats and IBS

Cold, pressed, unrefined nut or seed oil like flaxseed, walnut or pumpkin seed oils contain the essential fatty acids omega-6 linoleic acid and omega-3 alpha-linolenic acid. In the body, omega-3 and omega-6 oils are converted into prostaglandins, essential for their inflammatory-reducing properties and for healthy colon function.

The best seeds and oils for essential fats are flax, linseeds, pumpkin, hemp, sunflower, safflower, sesame, corn, walnut, soya bean and wheatgerm. Take the oil daily on salads or in other dishes. The oil loses critical nutrients when heated, so make sure you consume it cold. Cold-water fish oils from salmon and mackerel are another good source for essential fatty acids. For best results, eat fish and a salad with a dressing of unrefined, cold-pressed sunflower or walnut oils. The fatty acid of the fish helps to ensure the conversion of the oil's linoleic acid to colon-friendly prostaglandins.

Adjusting your eating habits

Healthy eating is the first step. The second step is to start adjusting your eating habits according to the guidelines below. If you haven't tried these food-related suggestions yet, they really are worth a shot as some people (but not all – remember, we don't really know what causes IBS, so there is no magic bullet for IBS; what works for one person may not work for another) have found them to be the answer.

1 Keep a food journal

Record everything you eat and drink for at least ten days and try to work out how your diet relates to your symptoms, by comparing what you have eaten with bad attacks. Write down everything you eat and drink and every symptom you experience (such as abdominal pain, diarrhoea, wind, bloating and so on), how long it lasts, and how severe it is. Try to write down too how much you eat, where and how you eat, how long it took you to eat your meal, and also what mood you are in when you eat. For example, did you eat a full plate of food? Did you eat on the move? Did you feel relaxed when you were eating? Becoming aware of what foods and eating habits may be triggering attacks can help you avoid that food and situation and find alternatives. Bear in mind that it is normal to have contractions of the colon about 30 to 60 minutes after a meal. The box below offers some suggestions on how to keep a food diary.

How to keep a food diary

Use a small notebook that you can carry with you and keep handy. Organize each page into columns. This can be done by using one page for each meal/snack, one page per day, or whatever works best for you (and the size of your notebook!).

The first column is 'How much?' Estimate the size (inches), weight (ounces), volume (cups) or number (e.g. 5) of the food you ate.

The second column is 'What kind?' What kind of food did you eat? Be very specific, and be sure to remember condiments and toppings such as butter, salad dressings, mayonnaise, etc.

The third column is 'Time'. What time of day did you eat the food?

The fourth column is 'Where?' Write down where you ate – in a restaurant, at the dining-room table, over the sink, in your car, etc.

The fifth column is 'Who?' Fill in who you were eating with, or whether you were alone.

The sixth column is for 'Activity'. Write down what you were doing while you ate. Were you working, driving, watching television, doing homework, etc.?

The seventh column is for your 'Mood'. Take notes on how you

---

were feeling while you were eating. Were you happy, sad, angry, stressed, etc.?

The eighth, and probably the most important, column is for 'Symptoms'. Write down any symptoms you may have experienced after you ate. Some examples might be diarrhoea, stomach upset, bloating, wind or heartburn.

Be honest! It's important to report everything (even those crisps you ate at 1 a.m.!).

Update your records as you eat during the day. It can be difficult to remember everything you ate if you only make entries once each day.

Be specific. The way a food was prepared or what it was served with can be important. For example, roast potatoes is a better description than just 'potatoes'.

Stick with it! You may be amazed at how a simple journal can help you and your doctor with your treatment.

2 Avoid IBS trigger foods

One of the fundamental principles behind healing IBS via your diet is to avoid foods that trigger or irritate a spastic colon via the gastro-colic reflex that occurs when food enters the stomach, and to eat foods that soothe and regulate the colon.

Please don't read this list and think you can never eat any of these foods again. Although they are all IBS triggers and some of them may need to be eliminated from your diet, others can still be eaten as long as you follow the 'how to eat' guidelines for IBS below. Try not to think of this as the beginning of a diet, but the beginning of a healthier way of eating.

Common IBS triggers

- Red meat (minced beef, hamburgers, hot dogs, steaks, roast beef, pastrami, salami, bologna, pepperoni, corned beef, ham, bacon, sausage, pork chops, and anything else that comes from cows, pigs, sheep, goats, deer, etc.).
- The dark meat and skin of poultry (skinless white meat is fine, as is seafood, and try to buy organic turkey and chicken).
- Dairy products (cheese, butter, sour cream, cream cheese, milk, cream, half-and-half, ice cream, whipped cream, yogurt, frozen yogurt). Even if you are not lactose intolerant, dairy products can

be an IBS trigger food. It's not the lactose, but the high fat content of most dairy products that can cause symptoms. Even skimmed, semi-skimmed and lactose-free dairy foods can trigger IBS attacks. In addition to fat and lactose, dairy products contain components such as the proteins whey and casein, which can cause severe digestion problems.

- Saturated fat. The gut normally responds to food by contracting, and the strength of the response seems to be linked to the amount of saturated fat in the meal. So try to cut down on the saturated fat in your diet. Avoid saturated fat-rich food, such as dairy food, red meat and egg yolks, and ensure your milk is skimmed or semi-skimmed, cook with minimal fat by baking or steaming food rather than frying or roasting, and choose monosaturated fats found in olive oil, canola oil, peanut oil, peanuts, cashews and almonds. Other high-in-saturated-fat foods to watch out for are: butter; peanut butter; chips/french fries; tartar sauce; salad dressings; onion rings; all oils, fats, spreads, etc.; fried chicken; anything battered and deep-fried; anything skillet-fried in fat of any kind; shortening; margarine; mayonnaise; olives; nuts and nut butters; croissants, pastries, biscuits, scones and doughnuts; pie crust; potato chips (unless they are baked); corn chips and nachos (unless they're baked); store-bought dried bananas (they're almost always deep fried); solid chocolate (baking cocoa powder is fine); solid carob (carob powder is fine). Watch out too for hidden sources of saturated fat found in biscuits, crackers, pancakes, waffles, scones, pastries, doughnuts, and mashed potatoes.

The thought of giving up these foods may seem shocking at first, but if you give it a go you'll be surprised how easy it can actually be, especially nowadays when there are so many fat-free products and healthy, tasty substitutes that will let you cook and eat safely while still enjoying many of your traditional favourite foods. And whenever you're tempted to indulge in a high-risk treat, remind yourself that the enjoyment quickly disappears when it's followed by a vicious IBS attack.

GI irritants

In addition to saturated fats, the following can also be dangerous. If they trigger an attack, the solution is simple: avoid them and find healthier, safer alternatives:

Coffee, both regular and decaffeinated, contains an enzyme that is an extremely powerful GI tract irritant. Start cutting back today and drink herbal teas instead. Coffee, and tea, also contains caffeine which is a GI stimulant and should be avoided, especially in higher doses.

Chocolate, sweets and cakes are high in saturated fat. When you fancy something sweet, there are alternatives. See the display box for alternatives.

Sweet alternatives

If you're craving sweets, your healthiest alternative is to go for fresh or dried fruits such as apricots, apples or pears. Fruit is power packed with antioxidants and nutrients that can give you a natural energy boost.

As long as you can tolerate dairy foods, unsweetened low-fat live yoghurt mixed with fruit (or a spoonful of low-fat jam now and again) is a sweet, creamy, satisfying, nutritious and light alternative to sugary, fatty cakes and desserts that will weigh you down.

Instead of guzzling a soda loaded with sugar, additives and calories, try a smoothie instead. Smoothies are made from the juice of real fruits. They are scrumptious, sweet and full of goodness.

Try a bowl of hot oat cereal with a pinch of stevia or maple syrup on top. It will satisfy your sweet tooth, keep hunger at bay, and give you a comfort fix at the same time. Stevia is a herb that is 300 times sweeter than sugar, with negligible calories. Use it sparingly in cooking or for sprinkling on cereals and desserts.

A small bar of good-quality dark chocolate is naturally rich in health-boosting flavonoids. In moderation it can offer chocoholics a healthy, low-fat alternative to high-fat, high-sugar chocolate bars.

Alcohol is a GI irritant and often triggers IBS attacks, especially on an empty stomach (though small amounts of alcohol used in cooking are fine). At the time of writing, no studies have proven that alcohol either instigates or worsens these conditions, but drinking has been proven to have significant effects on the digestive system as well as the rest of the body. Many people with IBS find that an occasional drink does not worsen their condition, but some may discover (as with other foods and drinks through trial and error) that it does have a detrimental effect. Additionally, the effect of alcohol on the liver, the stomach and overall health should be weighed against the positive effects, as well as the importance of social drinking on quality of life.

Carbonation in soda drinks, cola and mineral water can cause bloating and cramps.

Artificial sweeteners, particularly sorbitol, can trigger pain, cramps, wind, bloating and diarrhoea.

Artificial fats, namely olestra (Olean), can cause abdominal cramping and diarrhoea in people who don't even have IBS – imagine what it can do to you.

MSG (monosodium glutamate) is a food additive that has been linked to all sorts of digestive upsets. It can simply be avoided by insisting that your food and take-away meals are MSG free.

Avoid *chewing gum*, as it causes you to swallow excess air, which can trigger problems.

3 Supplement with essential fatty acids (EFAs)

While you should steer clear of saturated fats, healthy fats are essential and necessary. This is because your body, in particular your heart, needs healthy fats in order to function so you should never go on a fat-free diet. Instead, keep your fat intake to 20–25 per cent of your total calories, and make your fats count. As mentioned above in the healthy eating guidelines, the fats you include in your diet should be monounsaturated and contain the essential fatty acids omega-3 and omega-6, so choose fat sources such as olive oil, canola oil, avocados, nuts, seeds, fatty fish, flax oil, etc.

It's especially important to have a high intake of omega-3 and omega-6 because both create prostaglandins – hormone-like substances that help produce healthy cardiovascular, immune, nervous and reproductive systems. Although omega-3 contains more linolenic acid than omega-6 fats, both also contain important health-boosting substances. There are thousands of other reasons to make sure your diet is rich in omega oils, but in the case of IBS, eating plenty of cod, herring, mackerel, sardines and salmon, or supplementing with flaxseed oil if you don't eat fish, may boost your digestion.

(*Note*: Because all fats, even heart-healthy choices, are still potential IBS triggers, please follow the dietary guidelines detailed in the 'watch how you eat' section below.)

4 Fill up on soluble fibre

While fats and GI irritants are best reduced or completely eliminated from your diet, there's another crucial component to eating safely for IBS: understanding the difference between soluble and insoluble fibre. Soluble fibre can help both constipation and diarrhoea, but insoluble fibre can make diarrhoea worse. Those who suffer from diarrhoea should increase the amount of fibre they get from soluble fibre found in oat bran or psyllium (natural vegetable fibre) which is available in over-the-counter supplements.

For many people with IBS, soluble fibre is the single most important dietary aid, but soluble fibre is not typically found in foods most people think of as 'fibre', such as bran or raw leafy green vegetables. Soluble fibre is actually found in foods commonly thought of as 'starches', though soluble fibre itself differs from starch as the chemical bonds that join its individual sugar units cannot be digested by enzymes in the human GI tract. In other words, it passes through your body intact.

Good sources of soluble fibre

- Rice.
- Pasta and noodles.
- Oatmeal.
- Barley.
- Fresh white breads such as French or sourdough (*not* wholewheat or wholegrain).
- Rice cereals.
- Flour tortillas.
- Soya products.
- Quinoa.
- Corn meal.
- Potatoes.
- Carrots.
- Yams.
- Sweet potatoes.
- Turnips.
- Rutabagas.
- Parsnips
- Beets.
- Squash and pumpkins.
- Mushrooms.
- Chestnuts.

- Avocados (though they do have some fat).
- Bananas.
- Apple sauce.
- Mangoes.
- Papayas (also digestive aids that relieve wind and indigestion).

5 Eat insoluble fibre with caution

Insoluble fibre foods, such as wholegrains, figure strongly in a healthy diet, but if you've got IBS they need to be eaten with caution because, like saturated fat, they can trigger symptoms. Unlike saturated fat, however, you cannot simply minimize your insoluble fibre intake, as this will leave you with nutritional deficiencies. The solution is to eat insoluble fibre foods with caution, and you'll be able to enjoy a wide variety of them, in very healthy quantities, without a problem:

- Wholewheat flour, wholewheat bread, wholewheat cereals.
- Wheat bran.
- Wholegrains, wholegrain breads, wholegrain cereals.
- Green beans.
- Granola.
- Muesli.
- Seeds.
- Nuts.
- Popcorn.
- Beans and lentils (if mashed or pureed they're much safer).
- Berries (blueberries, strawberries, blackberries, cranberries, etc.).
- Peaches, nectarines, apricots, and pears with their skins on (when peeled they're much safer).
- Apples (when peeled they're safe).
- Rhubarb.
- Melons.
- Oranges, grapefruits, lemons, limes.
- Dates and prunes.
- Grapes and raisins.
- Cherries.
- Pineapple.
- Greens (spinach, lettuce, kale, collards, watercress, etc.).
- Whole peas, snow peas, snap peas, pea pods.
- Sweetcorn.

- Bell peppers (roasted and peeled they're safer).
- Celery.
- Onions, shallots, leeks, scallions, garlic.
- Cabbage, bok choy, Brussels sprouts.
- Broccoli.
- Cauliflower.
- Tomatoes.
- Cucumbers.
- Sprouted seeds (alfalfa, sunflower, radish, etc.).
- Fresh herbs.

The secret is not to eliminate these foods completely, but to eat them with a larger quantity of soluble fibre. For example, you can stir-fry veggies into fried rice or blend fresh fruit into a smoothie to drink after a breakfast bowl of oatmeal. For fruits, vegetables, and legumes in general, peeling, chopping, cooking and pureeing them will significantly minimize the impact of their insoluble fibre. It's also best to avoid eating insoluble fibre foods on an empty stomach, and to eat them cooked or made into soups and sauces rather than whole and raw. For beans and lentils, cook and blend them into sauces, dips, soups or spreads. For nuts, finely grind and incorporate them into breads or cakes with white flour, which gives a safe soluble fibre base. For bran and other wholegrains, eat them in small quantities following soluble fibre. For raw fruit and green salads, eat them at the end of a soluble-fibre meal instead of at the beginning.

Problem fruits and vegetables

The following fruits and vegetables can be particularly troublesome for IBS:

- *Sulphur-containing foods* (garlic, onions, leeks, broccoli, cauliflower, cabbage, asparagus and Brussels sprouts). In addition to their high amounts of insoluble fibre, these also produce significant gas in the GI tract and this can trigger attacks. As with all other fruits and veggies, they are extremely nutritious foods which should not be eliminated from your diet, simply treated with caution.
- *Acidic foods* (citrus fruits, vinegars and cooked tomatoes) should be treated with caution too as their acidity can trigger symptoms. Once again, follow the rules for insoluble fibre and eat these foods in smaller quantities incorporated with soluble fibre – but make sure you eat them.
- *Fructose*, a fruit sugar found in honey and fruit juice, can cause wind, bloating and diarrhoea, so it is best to eat this in small amounts along with soluble fibre.

If you have days when almost everything you eat seems to trigger an attack you need to avoid insoluble-fibre foods completely, restrict your diet to soluble fibre foods only, and to give your stomach a rest.

6 Keep your fibre intake below 30 grams a day

Some people are so keen to increase their fibre intake that they take it way over the limit of 30 grams a day without realizing it. Ideally, you should balance your fibre intake from both soluble and insoluble fibre sources to between 22 and 28 grams a day. The reason that fibre helps is that it absorbs water from the intestines and keeps moisture in the stool, thus preventing constipation. Fibre also fills out your colon with a bulking effect that can help prevent diarrhoea and painful spasms. The trouble is that there is a fine line between too much and too little fibre, and if you eat too much fibre this can cause excessive bowel movements, bloating and wind. However, don't let this steer you away from increasing your fibre intake. The only way to find out if fibre can help is to give it a try. Bear in mind that it is normal to have some bloating and wind in the first few weeks of a fibre-rich diet, so stick with it for a week or two. If things don't improve, you need to ease up on the fibre and try a different approach.

7 Watch how you eat

Diet can help or hurt IBS, based on how different foods physically affect your digestive system. However, it's not just what you eat that counts – it's also *how* you eat.

First of all, eating smaller meals through the day is important. Smaller meals are easier on your already stressed digestive system. Eating four to six small meals and snacks throughout the day will help your stomach and ease your symptoms. Snacking on small amounts of food throughout the day will keep you from getting ravenous and then over-eating, which can overload your digestive system and trigger an attack. Eating little and often and never allowing more than three hours between a meal or snack has another benefit; it allows you to treat yourself to the occasional indulgence. This is because if your stomach is well stabilized by a recent intake of soluble fibre you can afford the odd bar of chocolate or slice of cake.

Second, make sure you take your time when you eat, and chew your food thoroughly. Eating quickly encourages you to swallow too much air which can cause problems, and food that hits your stomach without being chewed properly further stresses your digestive system. The message is simple: take your time when you eat.

Third, if you are addicted to junk food, fast food, food that is highly processed and refined, and tend to rely on ready-prepared meals instead of cooked ones, this is going to play havoc with your digestive system. Try to stick with foods that are as natural as possible, and as much as possible prepare your meals from scratch. This is nutritionally sound advice, whether you have IBS or not!

And finally, it goes without saying that gulping your food down quickly, eating on the move, arguing or feeling anxious while you eat will all play havoc with your digestive system. The calmer and happier you are when you eat, the more likely you are to digest it well. (See Chapter 7: Healing IBS with stress management.)

A typical meal plan for those with IBS

Breakfast. A bowl of high-fibre wholewheat cereal such as untoasted muesli or oat porridge with fresh or tinned fruit and reduced-fat milk or calcium-fortified soya milk and/or wholemeal or wholegrain toast with minimal margarine and jam or Vegemite. Herbal tea.

Lunch. Sandwiches made with wholemeal bread with low-fat cheese, lean turkey, tinned fish and lashings of salad. Tinned or fresh fruit with low-fat yoghurt. Water, herbal tea or diluted juice.

Main evening meal. Lean grilled chicken with lemon juice and pepper. Served with salad, boiled new potatoes or baked potato and wholemeal bread.

Snacks. You can spread snacks throughout the day – fresh fruit, low-fat yoghurt, and low-fat wheat crackers with low-fat cheese, frozen yogurt, pretzels, wholegrain rice, wholewheat toast, or low-fat bran muffin. Water, tea or diluted juice.

The seven golden rules of the IBS diet

1 Eat soluble fibre whenever your stomach is empty, and make soluble-fibre foods the biggest part of every meal and snack.
2 Aim to eat 22–28 grams, but no more than 30 grams, of fibre a day.
3 Never eat saturated fat on an empty stomach and without soluble fibre.
4 Eliminate as much as possible all red meat, dairy, fried foods, egg yolks, coffee, soda pop and alcohol from your diet.
5 Make sure you get enough essential fats (or EFAs) and healthy protein every day.

6 Eat little and often and don't leave more than three hours between meals and snacks.

7 Take time to savour and enjoy your food.

For healthy eating adjustments for specific symptoms, such as constipation and diarrhoea, see Chapter 9: A to Z of specific symptoms and natural ways to beat them.

Eating out if you've got IBS

Eating out at restaurants or social functions can be tough if you've got IBS. It is especially trying when you are dining with people you have a professional relationship with, or hope to date, since they are not likely to know about your health problems. So how do you handle eating out without bringing attention to your problem?

Tips for enjoyable eating out

Have a plan of attack

Before you leave for the restaurant, decide on what you will eat and how much you will eat. If you're afraid that you will be hungry and tempted to eat something you shouldn't, then have a safe snack before you leave. If you know where you're going, phone the restaurant beforehand and ask about the menu. Many restaurants and catering venues also have webpages that include their menus.

Check out the loos first

Ask the host or hostess where the loos are located before you sit down to eat, or right after being shown to your table. If your dining companions don't know about your health problems, you can use the excuse of wanting to wash your hands before dinner. This way, you know where the facilities are located and you can check to be sure they're clean and stocked.

Skip the cocktails

Alcoholic drinks may not be a good idea for people with IBS. Try sparkling water or a virgin cocktail instead.

Ask your server

Don't be afraid to ask your server how a food is prepared or if it can be prepared in a 'lean' way, not a fried or creamy way. Ask for tomato sauce rather than cream sauce and look for menu items that are prepared in low-fat ways – baked, boiled, char boiled, barbecued, stir-fried, poached, roasted, grilled, steamed and braised. Always ask for salad dressing on the side. For dessert, choose frozen yogurt, sorbet and fruit salad.

Watch the appetizers

Appetizers such as mozzarella sticks, hot wings, nachos and chicken fingers are all fatty, fried or dairy-filled foods that might not be good to your colon. If everyone else is having an appetizer and you're feeling left out, have some soup instead or dig into the bread basket.

Anticipate any awkward questions

If someone asks you why you are requesting a certain dish to be cooked in a particular way, you could mention your illness briefly but if you prefer not to, then 'I'm on a diet' or 'I stopped eating red meat and dairy products' are also common reasons to give that aren't likely to raise more questions.

Vegetarianism and IBS

Laura, 54, describes how a close examination of her diet helped her IBS: 'I was placed on every kind of medication, and sometimes they worked in the short term, sometimes they didn't work at all. The doctor finally suggested trying to alter my diet in cycles, and we discovered that eating meat was my problem. I became a vegetarian and no longer have constant problems. Sometimes I even go years without any pain at all. It's worth all the effort you put into it when you finally feel better.'

A well-planned vegetarian diet that includes plenty of healthy protein closely corresponds to healthy eating principles for IBS in terms of fat, carbohydrate and fibre content. Vegetarian diets tend to be low in saturated fat and animal protein and to contain sufficient fibre, all of which have been shown to be beneficial for IBS. The only danger for vegetarians is that their diet becomes too high in fibre – that is, more than 30 grams a day. This will result in a worsening of IBS symptoms with bloating, wind, abdominal pain and diarrhoea.

Weight loss if you've got IBS

Can you lose weight when you are trying to keep your IBS symptoms under control with diet? The short answer to this question is yes, absolutely! The IBS diet guidelines given above are very compatible with weight loss because they are nutrient-rich, low-fat, plant-based and incorporate plenty of fibre.

Common sense rules of regular meals, smaller meals, mindful eating and regular physical activity (more about the amazing benefits of exercise if you've got IBS is included in Chapter 7) are great guidelines for both digestive and overall health. If you're feeling daunted by trying to manage your IBS through diet and to lose weight at the same time, the following case history may inspire you:

Lucy, 42

To celebrate the New Year I decided to take my partner, Steve, on a combination business/pleasure trip to Paris, as it's such a beautiful city. When we got on the plane I couldn't get the seatbelt around me, however, and had to ask the skinny flight attendant for an extension.

We had barely got off the plane when I became ill. My stomach hurt so much that it made the rest of my body ache. I was bloated, nauseous, and had cold sweats. All I wanted to do was to break wind, but I couldn't. We had planned to have dinner that evening with some colleagues. Steve went, but I spent the entire evening leaving the table every 10 or 15 minutes to go and sit on the loo and cry. Each time I returned, the table would fall silent and all eyes would be on me out of concern. It was very embarrassing.

That was the straw that broke the camel's back. I vowed to myself that I was going to do something about my weight and my IBS. I could not, would not, continue to live like this. Spending all my spare time on the toilet or on the couch in pain, never wanting to do anything, was just too much.

I must admit, I was not eating properly. I would have espresso and pastries for breakfast, cheeseburger with chips or fried chicken for lunch, an espresso frappuccino on the way home, pizza or other fast food for dinner, and who knows what for snacks and dessert. I probably drank four to six cans of coke a day. When all was said and done, I was easily consuming 4,000 calories a day of rubbish!

I went on the internet and read some books and started to learn about IBS and how food can both help and hinder. I cleaned out the cupboards, donated foods that were not safe or healthy for me to eat to a local food bank, and stopped drinking caffeine. Now I drink lots of water, tea and the occasional sports drink. (I do OK with those, but some people don't.) I'm also starting eating little and often and watching my intake of saturated fat.

I started going to the gym after work for just 15 to 20 minutes. Slowly that increased to 30, 40, 50 and even 60+ minutes! My weight loss wasn't dramatic at first, just one or two pounds a week, but my doctor told me that this was the safest and most healthy way to lose weight and keep it off. He was right. By the end of the year I was down to a size 14 and I haven't been that size for years. My diet and lifestyle changes have added a good ten years to my life, and I feel that I'm living again. I never feel hungry because the next snack or meal is only an hour or two away and the food I'm eating is tasty and satisfying and even allows me the odd bar of chocolate. Even my sex drive has increased. I can't say enough how very important it is to take charge of your diet and get some kind of exercise! Even if it is just a walk around the block every day, it's a start! I have only called in sick to work for IBS-related issues once in the last year, and it is wonderful to be able to walk around my neighbourhood without sweating and being out of breath or wondering where the nearest loo is.

5

Healing IBS with supplements

Many people with IBS have found supplements to be a better, safer and more effective option than drugs and medical treatments.

Sally, 27
I tried taking digestive enzymes with acidophilus and found significant relief within three days. I am not afraid to eat now, but find that I still cannot eat very much refined sugar or high-fibre vegetables. I have also added a cup or two per day of peppermint and chamomile tea. When I do have an episode it occurs late in the day and by the next morning I am feeling back to normal.

Austin, 44
I used to get bouts of painful diarrhoea. What has helped me for more than two years is calcium carbonate, an over-the-counter supplement. I take three tablets a day, one at each meal. The only side-effect is at the beginning of taking the calcium you may have some wind or indigestion, but this usually goes away after taking a regular dose for a few days.

Laura, 40
After about six months of a horrendously restrictive diet (ultra low-fat vegan with no raw veggies or fruit except bananas) and a lot of Metamucil [a fibre supplement], I managed to get it partly under control. But if I deviated from the diet, the chronic diarrhoea would come back. Someone I met told me that she had helped her IBS by taking a tablespoonful of freshly ground linseeds with a glass of water or juice every morning. I thought it was another crackpot cure, but eventually I decided to try it. She had told me that pre-ground linseed didn't work because linseed starts to oxidize as soon as you grind it and that whole linseeds are no good either, because they cannot be digested properly. After years of IBS, in about two weeks it just went away. I cannot believe that I now have perfectly normal, regular bowel movements.

Recent surveys indicate that more than half of people with IBS use supplements and alternative therapies (see the next chapter) to seek relief. Listed below are the many types of supplements for IBS, which can be very effective. In particular, soluble-fibre supplements, herbs (such as peppermint and fennel) that have beneficial effects on the GI tract, probiotics, calcium and/or magnesium, and digestive enzymes are the most popular supplements with proven benefit. Results are usually felt very quickly – sometimes even immediately.

There is no guarantee that any of the herbs or supplements discussed here will help you, but if you decide you want to experiment it's a good idea to make an appointment with a herbalist and/or nutritionist first. This is because, as stressed previously, your IBS symptoms and triggers are unique to you. If you are taking medication, are pregnant or hoping to be so, you should also consult your doctor before taking any supplements.

Mineral supplements

If diarrhoea is one of your symptoms, the chances are you will have lost many vital vitamins and minerals. Calcium is often the mineral most recommended by doctors, but other important minerals include magnesium and zinc.

Calcium

Most of us think of calcium as a mineral important for bones and teeth, but it has many other vital functions. Calcium is important for a healthy heart, normal nerve function and muscle function. (Together with magnesium, it provides the mechanism for muscle contraction and relaxation.) Calcium also activates enzymes, promotes cell division, allows the transport of nutrients through cell membranes, and plays a role in iron utilization.

If you have IBS and are concerned about your calcium intake but can't tolerate dairy products, you can try other sources of calcium than milk and cheese. These sources include broccoli, spinach, turnip greens, tofu, yogurt, sardines and salmon with bones, calcium-fortified milk and breads, calcium supplements, and some antacid tablets. For best absorption, calcium supplements should be taken with food, and doses should not exceed 500 milligrams at a time.

Magnesium

Magnesium deficiency is very common today as there is little magnesium in the soil, what little magnesium is found in food is lost during cooking and processing, and most of us simply do not eat enough magnesium-rich foods, which include wholegrains, dark green vegetables, nuts and seeds.

Calcium is important, but without magnesium calcium cannot function. This is because magnesium works in synergy with calcium. If there is too much calcium and not enough magnesium, you can get aches and pains and fatigue. Because magnesium is crucial for carbohydrate metabolism which creates energy, fatigue is in fact one of the first symptoms of magnesium deficiency. In terms of GI tract function, calcium has a constipating effect, whereas magnesium acts as a laxative. As a result, calcium supplements can be truly beneficial for people with diarrhoea-predominant IBS, and magnesium supplements can work wonders for IBS constipation.

To take a calcium/magnesium supplement that will keep your bowel function in balance, it is typically recommended to use a 2:1 ratio of calcium to magnesium, as many people absorb magnesium more easily than calcium. Be careful that you do not exceed the recommended daily amounts of calcium (1,000 milligrams) and magnesium (400 milligrams).

Magnesium supplements come in many forms. Magnesium oxide has laxative effects which can be useful for constipation, but powdered forms of magnesium citrate are better for diarrhoea.

Zinc

Zinc is an essential trace mineral, which means that it must be obtained from the diet since the body cannot make enough. Low zinc levels have been reported in people with IBS. Zinc plays an important role in the immune system, which may explain why it is helpful in protecting against infections such as colds. Zinc also plays a role in the regulation of appetite, stress levels, taste and smell. Deficiencies in zinc can play a role in chronic diarrhoea. The best food sources of zinc for people with IBS are legumes (especially lima beans, black-eyed peas, pinto beans, soya beans, peanuts), miso, tofu, brewer's yeast, cooked greens, mushrooms, green beans, tahini, and pumpkin and sunflower seeds. Red meat and wholegrains are also sources of zinc, but they are also potential irritants, so supplementation might be wise. Zinc sulphate is the most frequently used supplement, but it is also the least easily absorbed and may cause stomach upsets. Healthcare providers usually prescribe 220 milligrams of zinc sulphate, which contains approximately 55 milligrams of elemental zinc. The more easily absorbed forms of zinc are zinc picolinate, zinc citrate, zinc acetate, zinc glycerate, and zinc monomethionine. If zinc sulphate causes stomach irritation, another form, such as zinc citrate, should be tried.

Vitamin supplements

The main recommended vitamins for people with IBS are Vitamins A, D, E and K because they are not as easily absorbed as water-soluble vitamins are and, like calcium and magnesium, they are likely to be drained out of the body by diarrhoea.

Vitamin A

Good food sources of Vitamin A include dark green leafy vegetables, fruits, dairy foods and eggs. Cod liver oil is the main supplement source.

Vitamin D

The main source of Vitamin D is sunshine, and people who live in northern climates need extra Vitamin D from cod liver oil, Vitamin D-fortified cereals and fish oils.

Vitamin E

Vitamin E, like Vitamin A, is a powerful antioxidant that protects your body from ageing and disease-promoting free radical damage. Food sources of Vitamin E include vegetable oils, nuts and green leafy vegetables.

Vitamin K

This is responsible for blood clotting and is found in green leafy vegetables.

Taking a vitamin and mineral supplement

Diet should always be the foundation stone, but if you have IBS and find it hard to eat a balanced diet, a combined vitamin and mineral supplement will act as an important nutritional insurance. There is also some research that suggests that food sensitivity that can trigger symptoms of IBS is more likely if you are lacking certain vitamins and minerals. Always choose a supplement that has as many vitamins and minerals as possible, in particular calcium, magnesium, zinc, Vitamins A, C, D, E and K. Although there is no guarantee that this will improve your IBS, it will certainly help prevent nutritional deficiency and to improve your overall health. It may also help to prevent some of the common health problems linked with vitamin and mineral deficiency which include: poor immunity, fatigue, PMS, poor wound healing, nose bleeds, dry skin, dull hair, gum disease, mouth ulcers, cracked lips, sore tongue, constipation and feeling tired all the time.

Herbal healing

Anise

Anise contains an oil that helps gastric juice production and can prevent and treat GI cramping. Anise can be used to treat both constipation and diarrhoea because it helps to normalize bowel function. It is also a mild sedative and can ease stress and anxiety.

Artichoke leaf extract (ALE)

This may have potential for treating IBS. In a study evaluating the use of ALE in those people with dyspepsia or indigestion, a small group was identified as having IBS. This group of people with IBS had the severity of their symptoms reduced and provided an overall favourable evaluation of the extract. As many as 96 per cent of them claimed that the artichoke leaf extract was well tolerated and that it worked at least as well as other therapies used for their symptoms.

Caraway

This is a very safe herb that can aid digestion because it increases the production of gastric juices and is a natural antibiotic. Researchers have found that several chemicals in caraway can help to relax muscles in the intestines and help eliminate the gas that causes pain and wind.

Cat's claw

Cat's claw is a vine that grows in the rain forests of South America. In the villages of Peru, local medicine people have used cat's claw for hundreds of years to treat a wide variety of ailments, including stomach pain, ulcers, and other GI complaints. Modern research has found active ingredients in cat's claw that stimulate the immune system with a possible anti-viral effect. Cat's claw also neutralizes free radicals, the cell-damaging by-products of oxygen metabolism that contribute to inflammation. Cat's claw soothes irritated and inflamed tissues and helps to eliminate harmful organisms from the GI tract, making the herb potentially beneficial in IBS.

Chamomile

Research shows that chamomile can relieve GI stress by calming smooth muscle tissue, therefore relieving indigestion, bloating and wind. The only possible side-effect is an allergy to it as it is a member of the daisy family, which houses ragweed, a notorious allergen.

Evening primrose

Evening primrose oil (EPO) is rich in GLA, an essential fatty acid that keeps inflammation under control, supports immunity, and plays many other important roles. The human body can produce all but two fatty acids: omega-3 and omega-6 fatty acids. Both must be obtained through the diet or by the use of supplements. Obtaining a balance of these two fatty acids is essential. Essential fatty acids are needed for building cell membranes and are precursors for the production of hormones and prostaglandins. Modern diets tend to be lacking in quality sources of fatty acids.

Fennel

This liquorice-tasting herb can help to soothe the bowel by eliminating wind and bloating. It also helps to increase the production of gastric juices which can help digestion, normalize the contractions in the intestines and relieve abdominal pain. It is a natural bowel relaxant because it contains dopamine. Research in Germany has shown that fennel is safe for daily use and that it can be effective for abdominal pain, gas and bloating.

Ginger

Ginger isn't just helpful for nausea – it can also ease indigestion and gastrointestinal cramps because it can act as a strong digestive enzyme.

Grapefruit seed

Grapefruit seed extract is another herb that may benefit those who have IBS by keeping harmful organisms out of the intestinal tract (you can also eat the seed itself, though it is bitter!). Clinical and experimental studies indicate grapefruit seed extract has broad spectrum anti-microbial properties. Grapefruit seed extract also inhibits the growth of two ulcer-causing bacteria: *Helicobacter pylori* and *Campylobacter jejuni*. In one human study, grapefruit seed extract relieved constipation, wind and abdominal distress after four weeks.

Olive leaf

Olive trees are widely cultivated throughout Mediterranean countries for their universally popular fruit. But olive trees have more to offer than just the olive and its delicious, healthful oil. The olive leaf has been used as a traditional medicine in health conditions including malaria, infections, cardiovascular diseases, and for improving general well-being. Oleuropein, an active ingredient in olive leaf, shows promising anti-viral properties. Lab studies have found that oleuropein stimulates activity of immune cells called 'macrophages' which serve as the body's 'rubbish collectors' to remove toxins and destroy foreign organisms.

Oregano

The oils in oregano can help to relieve nausea, vomiting, diarrhoea and muscle cramps. They also increase gastric juice production and help to eliminate wind and bloating.

Peppermint oil

Peppermint is a favourite herb for relief of digestive problems such as upset stomachs, wind and colic in children. In Europe, peppermint oil is given routinely to people with IBS for its relaxing, soothing effect. Peppermint oil helps to relieve intestinal spasms. Its antispasmodic action has been demonstrated in laboratory animals. Peppermint oil relaxes the smooth muscle in the intestinal tract by acting as a mild 'calcium channel blocker' to reduce muscle contractions. Many clinical trials have shown that enteric-coated peppermint oil relaxes the intestine and relieves pain in people with IBS. Enteric-coated pills are recommended as they dissolve better in the intestines where they help to relax the muscles and relieve pain.

Other herbs that may play a role in digestive and intestinal health include bitter orange peel, areca seed and dandelion root. These are bitter herbs that can help to stimulate gastric juices, and they also increase the production of bile which helps to digest fats.

Digestive aids

One of the best ways to boost your digestion is to chew your food properly, but you may also want to consider taking some digestive aids to make sure that no incompletely digested food reaches your large intestine and triggers IBS symptoms. Digestive enzymes are best taken in the middle or towards the end of a meal and you should notice a difference in bloating and flatulence within 24 hours of taking them. Typically, digestive enzymes contain various combinations of the following ingredients:

- Amylase: for digesting carbohydrates in the small intestine.
- Betaine hydrochloric acid: for digestion in the stomach.
- Lipase: for fat digestion.
- Papaya and bromelaine: fruit sources for protein digestion.
- Pepsin: for protein digestion in the stomach.
- Peptidase: for protein digestion in the small intestine.

Probiotics

Probiotic supplements are designed to help maintain a healthy population of 'friendly' lactic acid-producing bacteria in the intestinal tract. ('Probiotic' means 'for life'.) Also known as 'friendly flora', these bacteria help to regulate elimination, support immunity in the gut, and keep 'unfriendly' bacteria such as *E. coli* in check. As we saw in Chapter 2, it is theorized that people with IBS may not have enough of these good bacteria. This possibility was tested in a study of 60 people with IBS who took either a lactobacillus supplement or a placebo daily for four weeks. Compared to those on placebo, those taking the probiotic had far less intestinal gas. Twelve months later, overall GI function remained better in the people who had received the bacteria supplement.

You'll find probiotics in live yogurt, but as yogurt isn't always a good choice if you've got IBS, you might want to try the capsule or powder form. Probiotic supplements should be taken with food. Researchers believe there may be hundreds of different kinds of good bacteria in the gut and, not surprisingly, there are many different kinds of probiotic supplements available. In supplement form you need to look for doses in the billions of cells. The range of the most common probiotic, Lactobacillus acidophilus, is from 1 to 10 billion active cells daily.

Soluble fibre supplements

Clinical studies have repeatedly proven the benefits of soluble fibre supplements for those with IBS. The United States Department of Agriculture (USDA) recommended minimum fibre intake for adults is 25 to 35 grams daily, and soluble fibre should account for one-third to one-half of this total amount. If you suffer from bouts of IBS constipation, you might want to take psyllium husk capsules or one to two tablespoonfuls of powder twice daily to maintain one or two bowel movements a day. Their effectiveness derives from a mucilate present in the seed husk that swells to between eight and fourteen times its original volume when mixed with water. In the intestines, psyllium forms a laxative bulk that gently scrubs the bowel and absorbs toxins.

Finding your winning formula

The supplements mentioned in this chapter have all been shown to be helpful for symptoms of IBS, and they may be helpful to you. Remember, though, that your IBS symptoms are as individual as you are and what works for one person may not work for you. You need to keep experimenting with your diet and with supplements until you find your own winning formula.

For more advice on supplements, see Chapter 9: A to Z of specific symptoms and natural ways to beat them.

(*Warning*: If you are pregnant, on medication, or suffer from any medical condition other than IBS, be sure to seek medical advice before experimenting with herbs and supplements.)

6

Healing IBS with complementary therapies

Complementary therapies can sometimes be of enormous help to people with IBS. Simon, for example, found relief with homeopathy and Fiona found that acupuncture eased her symptoms.

Fiona, 30

I have suffered for several years from what the doctors have diagnosed as irritable bowel syndrome. My IBS came on very suddenly, one evening, with severe abdominal pain. The pain was so intense that I began to hyperventilate. My husband rushed me to hospital where the doctors could find nothing wrong with me. They gave me morphine for the pain and sent me home.

I made several visits to different doctors, each one diagnosing IBS and suggesting eliminating the foods that cause pain, getting more exercise, and eliminating stress. They prescribed painkillers and muscle relaxants and sent me home feeling hopeless. The painkillers caused drowsiness and constipation, and the muscle relaxants caused my heart to race. I knew that I couldn't continue to use them, but really didn't want to anyway.

I wanted to find a natural way to combat this affliction. I took the doctors' advice and began walking to get my exercise. This seemed to help considerably, but I was unable to do it when in pain, as it made the pain much worse. I also eliminated the foods that seemed to bother me, such as cabbage, broccoli, corn, soda pop, and ice cream. I began taking acidophilus, a glass of prune juice every morning, and a calcium supplement; these all seemed to help relieve the pain and bouts of explosive diarrhoea to some degree, but not enough.

My son, who is studying complementary medicine, suggested I try homeopathy. I wasn't sure, but by this stage I was willing to give anything a try. I enjoyed the consultation as the homeopath didn't seem to be in such a hurry as most doctors I have seen and he wanted to know all about my diet and lifestyle. He urged me to continue with the dietary measures I had already taken, and to step up my stress management with some yoga. He also gave me a Colocynthis remedy and, within days of taking it, I felt so much better. Within weeks I wasn't getting the cramps any more and within months I had my energy back. I still have to be careful with what I eat and to watch my stress levels, but IBS isn't in control any more of my life, I am.

Simon, 31
I've suffered from IBS since I was 15 and have tried almost every supplement, complementary therapy and medication there is. Some work better than others but the only therapy I feel I can rely on 100 per cent is acupuncture. In the hands of a trained, experienced, licensed practitioner of traditional Chinese medicine, acupuncture has helped relieve my very painful symptoms time and time again. I am also taking a prescribed Chinese herbal formula consisting of tiny, inexpensive pills. And eureka! No more IBS problems.

The following complementary therapies listed in this chapter have helped people with IBS. Just as with traditional medicine and supplements for IBS, however, all treatments will not suit every person, so it is a matter of finding what works best for you. Remember too that your winning formula may not be a single approach, but a combination of approaches: diet, supplements, complementary therapies, stress management and consultation with your doctor.

(Warning: If you are pregnant, on medication or suffer from any medical condition other than IBS, be sure to seek medical advice first before experimenting with homeopathy, aromatherapy and Chinese herbal medicine.)

Healing with acupuncture

Acupuncture has its roots in ancient Chinese medicine, but has become popular worldwide for many ailments. The basic theory underlying acupuncture is that there are channels of energy (Qi), called meridians, that run through the body. On the meridians are 360 acupuncture points. In a state of good health, energy flows freely along these channels. In disease, the energy flow is disrupted, leading to symptoms. Acupuncture to specific points is thought to release the energy and redirect its flow. In some cases, electrical stimuli are given to the acupuncture needles to increase the effect (electro-acupuncture). Two very small trials examining acupuncture for the treatment of IBS have been performed with contradictory results. Despite this lack of data, many people pursue acupuncture for abdominal pain, bloating and nausea. Acupuncture is generally safe if performed by a licensed acupuncturist, and may be a good adjunct in those who are sensitive, intolerant or refractory to oral interventions. For severe cases, many acupuncturists will use acupuncture in conjunction with herbal therapy.

Acupressure is similar to acupuncture, but instead of inserting needles at selected points, the meridians are stimulated using firm thumb pressure or fingertip massage. The best-known example of acupressure is shiatsu massage.

Healing with aromatherapy

Massage of the stomach and lower back can often be helpful in getting a constipated bowel moving, relieving wind and distension, or easing pain associated with IBS. You can visit a qualified aromatherapist for a massage or you can do one yourself. You may also find it helpful to apply alternate hot and cold compresses to your abdomen first to stimulate circulation. (See box feature below.)

Therapeutic heat

Direct heat is a tremendously effective muscle relaxant, and can be wonderfully beneficial for most IBS symptoms. If you have access to a jacuzzi, steam bath or sauna, take advantage of this and try engaging in regular sessions of heat-induced bliss. A hot-oil massage, especially with aromatherapy, can work wonders too.

Make a particular effort to try heat therapy immediately before any upcoming stressful event. A simple hot bath will do, or even a long hot shower. You can also wrap yourself up in an electric blanket, or apply a hot water bottle, hot pack or heat wraps directly to your abdomen.

To make an aromatherapy massage oil you need a carrier oil, such as grapeseed. To one tablespoonful of the carrier oil you then add 10 to 20 drops of essential oil. Rosemary, chamomile and marjoram, separately or blended with oil of black pepper and fennel, are often recommended for IBS. Other essential oils are listed below:

- For constipation: black pepper, cardamom, fennel, ginger, lemon, peppermint, rosemary and sandalwood.
- For wind and bloating: cardamom, coriander, dill, peppermint.
- For diarrhoea: basil, chamomile, lemon, orange and peppermint.
- For abdominal pain: chamomile, clove, eucalyptus, ginger, lavender, neroli, peppermint, rosemary and thyme.

Once your oils are blending, you are ready for your massage:

1 Place the container of diluted oil in a bowl of warm water to gently heat it.
2 Lie down in a warm, quiet room and expose your abdomen.
3 Place some warmed oil on your hands and gently massage your abdomen. Work clockwise; start by the right side of your groin and massage with slow, circular movements, pressing deeply without causing discomfort. Work your way up to your ribcage, across your abdomen, and down the left side of your groin again. Your massage should last at least five minutes. You might find it easier to get a partner or friend to do this for you.

Traditional Chinese Medicine (TCM)

TCM is based on a holistic approach. Thus, a complete and proper diagnosis involves an analysis of parts of your whole body, other than your abdominal area. For instance, your practitioner may check your tongue to check for coating. He or she needs to do this to determine whether the coating on your tongue is related to your IBS systems. When you experience any pain or discomfort, as in the symptoms for IBS, TCM hypothesizes that your body is not in balance.

TCM uses a variety of different natural treatment methods to correct the imbalance. Chinese herbal medicine is one such method. Specific herbs are prescribed to treat specific symptoms that you are experiencing and to aid the body in healing. For example, if you experience bloating, then the herb that will be recommended to you is one that can help relieve the bloating.

An experienced TCM practitioner would be well versed in the herbs that can be used for your IBS treatment. However, as not all herbs for IBS treatment may be suitable, he or she will have to make sure that he recommends the right ones for your case. You will probably need to consume the herbal concoction a few times before you start to experience results. As in most natural treatments, TCM does require time for healing to take place.

Acupuncture (see above) is another natural IBS treatment that is part of TCM, and there are also TCM exercises like t'ai chi, yoga (see below) or qigong that you can do for relaxation and to still your mind. This helps to improve your overall well-being. Some people believe that using TCM as a natural IBS treatment option is a good idea, and there have been a limited number of research studies that suggest it may have positive benefits. Do, however, ensure that you get proper referrals for a good TCM practitioner before seeking a consultation.

Healing with homeopathy

Homeopathy works on the principle that a substance which in large doses will cause the symptoms of an illness can be used in minute doses to relieve the same symptoms. Treatments are prescribed according to your symptoms rather than the disease, so two people with IBS, having differing symptoms, would have different treatments. In the UK you are entitled to have homeopathic treatment on the NHS. Alternatively, you could consult a private homeopathic practitioner or buy remedies direct from a pharmacy. Although it is best to consult a specialist, you may find the following remedies helpful for specific symptoms. Your symptoms may initially get worse, but you need to persevere as this is often a sign that the remedy is working:

- Constipation with no desire to open the bowels: Alumina 6c.
- Constipation with spasm and an urge to open the bowels: Nux vomica 6c.
- Diarrhoea with nervousness and anxiety: Argentum 6c.
- Diarrhoea with flatulence and burning of the rectum: Aloe 6c
- Diarrhoea and foul-smelling stools: Sulphur 6c or podophyllum.
- Alternating diarrhoea and constipation: Argentum 6c or lilium tigrinum.
- Exhausting diarrhoea and flatulence: China 6c.
- Diarrhoea with abdominal pain: Arsenicum album 6c.
- Diarrhoea brought on by drinking coffee: Psorinum 6c.
- Cramping bowel pain: Colocynthis or Mag. Phos. 6c.
- Bloating and distension: Lycopodium 6c.
- IBS symptoms that are worse in the late afternoon and early evening: Lycopodium.
- IBS and extreme fatigue: Mag. Phos.
- An itching, burning rectum with oozing: Sulphur.

Healing with hypnotherapy

Hypnotherapy has been shown to be effective for IBS in several clinical trials. For example, in a review of 14 previous clinical studies published in the *American Journal of Clinical Hypnosis* in 2005 the conclusion drawn was that hypnotherapy produces consistently significant results in IBS.

Hypnotherapy usually requires weekly individual sessions over several months, but has been tried in groups and by self-instruction as well. It typically involves progressive relaxation followed by suggestions of soothing imagery and sensations focused on the individual's symptoms. Improvements in overall well-being, quality of life, abdominal pain, constipation and bloating have been noted. A hypnotherapist will take some background details about your IBS experiences and symptoms. Then he or she will coax you into a state of extreme relaxation, and take you through a programme of suggestion. For example, you may be asked to imagine that when you hold your hand over your stomach, a healing warmth is flowing into your abdomen, or you may be asked to visualize a fully working digestive system. You will remain in complete control of your actions at all times. A therapist may record each session on to audio cassette to allow you to maintain therapy between sessions and use the tape whenever the need is felt.

One of the difficulties with hypnosis is that it is very dependent on the therapist, and it may be difficult to find a therapist both trained in hypnosis and knowledgeable about functional GI disorders. Additionally, like many alternative therapies, it can be costly and often is not covered by insurance plans. If you are unable to attend regular sessions with a hypnotherapist or cannot afford the sessions, there are self-hypnosis programmes and cassettes designed to be used at home.

Movement therapy

No studies on IBS are available for specific movement therapies such as yoga or t'ai chi. It's been shown, however, that relaxation-response meditation aids symptoms of abdominal pain, bloating, flatulence and diarrhoea, based on a small study. These types of therapies are particularly attractive, as they have no potential worrying side-effects and may be helpful for symptoms outside the GI tract as well as promoting general stress reduction.

Yoga is a gentle movement therapy that uses posture, breathing techniques and relaxation to increase suppleness, calm the body and mind, and boost health and well-being. Like most therapies, it is best to learn from a qualified teacher who will be able to help you achieve mental control and the right yoga positions for you. Breathing plays a particularly important role in yoga as the breath is thought to embody the life force or prana. The following simple poses, which should be held for approximately 30 seconds at least once a day, are good examples of yoga positions that may benefit specific symptoms of IBS:

Constipation:
There are two positions that can help with this. The first is to lie flat on your back with your legs flat on the ground, and then slowly bring both your knees up into your chest. The second is the seated forward bend (see Figure 6.1) where you sit down with your back straight and your legs extended forward. You then gently lean forward as far as you can.

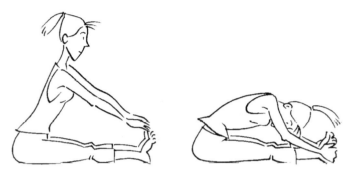

Figure 6.1   Seated forward bend

Diarrhoea:
Try the seated forward bend and the spinal twist (see Figure 6.2). For the spinal twist lie flat on your back with your legs flat on the ground. Slowly bring one leg into the chest and then twist it over the other leg so that it lies flat on the floor to your side.

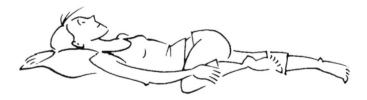

Figure 6.2   Spinal twist

Wind:
Try lying flat on your back and then bringing both knees into the chest. You could also try the relieving posture (see Figure 6.3) where you bring one leg into your chest and gently push it into your body with your arms.

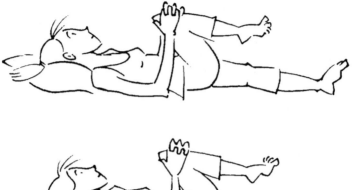

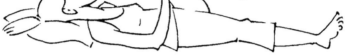

Figure 6.3   Relieving posture

Bloating:
For bloating, if you are very fit and flexible (and not in too much dis-comfort), try a shoulder stand. Another effective method is the arch and release technique (see Figure 6.4) whereby you 'stand' on your hands and knees and arch your back like a cat.

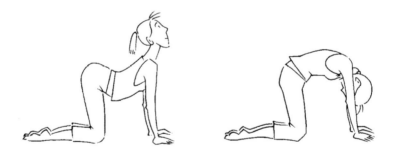

Figure 6.4   Arch and release (also known as cat and cow)

Indigestion:
Try the cobra and backward bend (see Figures 6.5 and 6.6). For the backward bend put your hands on your waist and gently tilt your shoul-ders, neck and head backwards as far as you can go without losing your balance. For the cobra lie flat on your stomach and gently arch up the upper part of your body, leaving your hips on the floor as you do so.

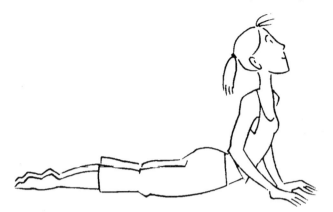

Figure 6.5 Cobra

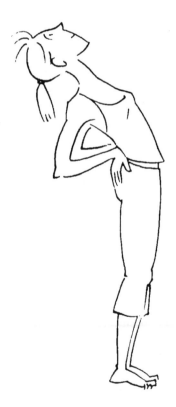

Figure 6.6 Backward bend

Reflexology

Reflexology is based on the theory that different 'reflux' zones on our feet correspond to other areas of our bodies. So, if one part of the foot is suffering from tension, that means that the corresponding part of the body is also suffering. The feet therefore form a kind of map of the body that can be used to treat symptoms.

By treating the problems in the foot, the body part will also be healed. Therapists may also treat your hands in a similar way. Reflexologists often say that stress and tension can be relieved by reflexology, but they also claim success with many other conditions, including digestive problems. In a reflexology session the therapist will take a background history and ask you questions about your symptoms. They will then treat you by applying pressure to various parts of your feet, and possibly hands as well. Treatment should not be painful, although it may be uncomfortable when areas of particular tension are massaged. Although there are no studies to prove that reflexology can be of benefit to people with IBS, some people with the condition have found it helpful as it can relieve fatigue and a number of stress-related symptoms such as tension, digestive problems and PMS.

If you are unable to visit a therapist, you and a partner or friend can easily learn how to give each other a foot massage by following the steps below:

- Soak feet in warm water for about ten minutes. You may wish to include drops of your favourite essential oil or bath salts. Peppermint or lavender oil is preferred by many. Make sure that your feet are completely dry before starting massage.
- Apply a moderate amount of cream or oil to the hands to add to comfort and ease. Make sure the hands are warm to avoid discomfort. Mineral oil is not absorbed in the skin, and it wipes off cleanly.
- Begin by stroking the top of the foot, and move in the direction from toe to ankle. Then continue by stroking the sole of the foot, first more gently, then by increasing pressure.
- Make circular motions with your thumb and fingers over the sole of the foot, and use more pressure in areas such as the heel or ball of the foot. Start from the top and work your way down. Do not neglect the sides.
- Holding the foot with one hand, use the other hand to rotate the foot, first at the ankle, and then near the ball of the foot. Be gentle. Repeat about five times in each direction.
- Knead the sole by holding the foot with one hand and making a fist

with the other, using moderate pressure into the sole. Give enough attention to the arch.

- Beginning with the big toe and working towards the little toe, take each toe individually. Roll the toe between your thumb and forefinger as you slide your fingers down the toe to the end, applying gentle pressure. Gently squeeze the end of each toe.
- Take your index finger and slide it between each toe about five times.
- To complete the massage, use your thumb and fingers to make the circular motions once again over the sole. End by stroking the sole and instep.
- Wipe off any excess cream or oil with a soft towel. Slip into thick socks to retain moisturizing, or slippers will suffice.
- Try to give equal attention to both feet, as the body abhors asymmetry.

7

Healing IBS with stress management

Victoria, 27
I feel my symptoms are connected with emotional problems and stress. Before I was diagnosed with IBS I used to think it was something I did to myself. I grew up with a father who verbally abused me. He would constantly shout at me when I was at the dinner table and this is when my abdominal pains started. I was never good enough for him and, although I worked hard to impress him, it seemed the harder I worked the more he shouted. In my late teens I started to avoid eating at the dinner table and eventually I didn't want to eat at all. Fortunately, around the same time my mother divorced my father and we moved away. I got some counselling and graduated from university with honours. I'm much happier now and am eating more or less normally again. My emotional problems are behind me, but I still find that when I'm under stress my IBS symptoms flare up.

Stress stimulates excessive adrenaline production, which in turn upsets the rhythmic muscle contractions of the gut. The stress response can also change the acid content of the stomach and in the body, killing the friendly bacteria needed for digestive harmony. Given that people with IBS are prone to suffer from irregular gut muscle contractions anyway, it's easy to see why stress can be such a powerful trigger or, in some cases, cause. Several interesting studies have actually shown the direct link between emotional stressors and subsequent IBS flares.

Fortunately, it's easy for the body to reverse its response to stress. Your body begins to relax as soon as your brain cancels signals to the central nervous system, and within about three minutes the panic messages cease and relaxation begins. Your body can't tell whether the relaxation response was triggered by a change in circumstances or attitude; either way, the symptoms are the same. So, just as stress can make IBS symptoms worse, reversing stress and learning how to relax may be able to ease symptoms.

An important part of the IBS healing plan is to learn techniques for reducing anxiety and stress. The techniques listed below can be helpful in promoting relaxation and minimizing stress-related IBS. Some can be learned in the time it takes to read this page, while others take a little more practice, but there's something here for everyone! With the exception of behavioural therapy, counselling and Reiki, they are all techniques you can try on your own.

Techniques to help relax your mind and your colon

Breathing

Most of us, especially when we are nervous or stressed, breathe rapidly and shallowly from the chest, but some people find that when they learn how to breathe from the diaphragm instead, it helps to promote relaxation. Deep breathing is an easy stress reliever that has numerous benefits for the body, including oxygenating the blood, which 'wakes up' the brain, relaxing muscles and quieting the mind. Breathing exercises are especially helpful because you can do them anywhere, and they work quickly so you can de-stress in a flash. The basic stress-relieving breathing exercise below is a great place to start.

Basic stress-relieving breathing exercise

- Sit or stand in a relaxed position.
- Slowly inhale through your nose, counting to five in your head.
- Let the air out of your mouth, counting to eight in your head as it leaves your lungs. Repeat several times. That's it!

TIPS

- As you breathe, let your abdomen expand outwards, rather than raising your shoulders. This is a more relaxed and natural way to breathe, and helps your lungs fill themselves more fully with fresh air, releasing more 'old' air.
- You can do this just a few times to release tension, or for several minutes as a form of meditation.
- If you like, you can make your throat a little tighter as you exhale so that the air comes out like a whisper. This type of breathing is used in some forms of yoga, and can add additional tension relief.

Behavioural therapy

One approach to coping with IBS is behavioural therapy. Why? Because stress and anxiety can worsen IBS symptoms, and behavioural therapy can help you cope with these feelings, thus reducing some IBS symptoms. It's not known what causes pressure and worry to trigger stomach pain, discomfort, diarrhoea or constipation. But learning how to manage emotional reactions effectively seems to prevent or ease suffering. Behavioural therapy helps people learn how to cope better with pain and discomfort, and how to relieve stressful situations in order to ward off severe IBS symptoms.

Unfortunately, behavioural therapy is not a cure-all. Some studies have shown the strategy does help to ease stress-related symptoms of IBS, but others show it does nothing for symptoms of constipation and constant stomach aches. Other studies show that it is best used with standard medical care. Before starting any form of therapy, talk with your doctor about how it may fit into your overall treatment plan. There are many different types of behavioural therapy. Here are techniques that have worked for some people with IBS:

Relaxation therapy

The goal is to get the mind and body in a calm, peaceful state. Techniques include meditation, progressive muscle relaxation (tensing and loosening individual muscles), guided imagery (visualization) and deep breathing.

Biofeedback

This strategy uses an electrical device to help people recognize their body's response to stress. Participants are taught, with the machine's help, to slow down their heart rate to a more relaxed state. After a few sessions, people are able to calm themselves down on their own.

Hypnotherapy

Participants enter an altered state of consciousness, either with a trained professional's help or on their own (after training). In this altered condition, visual suggestions are made to imagine pain going away. (See Chapter 6.)

Cognitive behavioural therapy

This is a form of psychotherapy that teaches you to analyse negative, distorted thoughts, and replace them with more positive and realistic thoughts.

Traditional psychotherapy

A trained mental health professional helps people to work out conflicts and understand feelings.

Counselling

Working with a counsellor to figure out how to cope with stress and IBS is one approach to living a more relaxed life. A study conducted through the department of medicine at Humboldt University in Berlin, and published in May 2002 in the *American Journal of Gastroenterology*, showed that when a segment of people with IBS attended ten sessions of therapy lasting one hour over a ten-week period, they felt more in control of their health and agreed that they had a better quality of life than those who did not partake in behavioural therapy. In the therapy sessions they were provided with information about IBS, as well as an analysis of their own unique symptoms and training in coping strategies and problem-solving. If counselling isn't an option, talking to loved ones or friends, or linking up with others with IBS via a support group or website, are other ways to ease stress.

Exercise

Whether you've got IBS or not, exercise is as important as a good diet for staying healthy both physically and emotionally. But are you doing it regularly? If you aren't, here are some very good reasons why you should.

Exercise firms your abdominal muscles and triggers intestinal contractions that keep your digestive system moving smoothly, which in turn helps with the passage of gas, reduces bloating and cramping, and results in more regular bowel movements. Exercise is also one of the best stress relievers.

Research shows that regular exercise can help relieve IBS symptoms, but you don't have to run a marathon to enjoy the benefits. As little as 30 minutes a day of light physical activity helps – for example, housework, walking the dog, climbing the stairs, mowing the lawn. And you don't have to do all your 30 minutes of activity at once either.

While at least 30 minutes of activity a day needs to be part of your IBS healing plan to fully enjoy all the benefits of exercise – lowered blood pressure and cholesterol level, weight loss and a reduction of anxiety and stress – you do have to work a bit harder with a well-rounded exercise programme. Research shows that people with IBS are less likely to exercise than people without it, so if you haven't been exercising regularly, then get started. The simple exercise tips below will show you that this isn't as exhausting or as complicated as it sounds.

Getting started with exercise

Most people can begin gradual, moderate exercise on their own. If you think there is a reason that you may not be able to exercise safely, talk to your doctor before beginning a new exercise programme. In particular, your doctor needs to know if you have heart trouble, high blood pressure or arthritis, or if you often feel dizzy or have chest pains.

In addition to increasing your activity levels during the day – for example, standing rather than sitting, getting off the bus a few stops early, taking the stairs instead of the lift, and so on – start off by exercising three or more times a week for between 5 and 15 minutes until you have gradually and slowly worked up to at least 30 minutes, four to six times a week. Getting to 30 minutes five times a week may take several weeks or even a few months to achieve, so don't worry if you feel exhausted after your first 10-minute session. Just stick with it and you'll soon find that your fitness levels and your enjoyment increase. If you don't think you can find a spare 30 minutes, try to include several short bouts of activity in a day, say three slots of 10 minutes. Exercising during a lunch-break or on your way to do errands may help you add physical activity to a busy schedule.

Choose an activity that you enjoy and one that you can start slowly and increase gradually as you become used to it. Walking is very popular and does not require special equipment. Other good exercises include swimming, biking and gentle trampoline. Exercise is any physical activity that raises the heart rate. You don't necessarily have to join a gym.

Start with an activity you can do comfortably. As a rule of thumb, when you are exercising you should be slightly out of breath but not so out of breath that you can't hold a conversation with someone. So if you find yourself panting, huffing and puffing, stop. You're exercising too hard.

Sample gentle exercise plan for walking, swimming, cycling and jogging

You should start your exercise session with a gradual warm-up period. During this time (about 5 to 10 minutes), you should slowly stretch your muscles first, and then gradually increase your level of activity. For example, begin walking slowly and then pick up the pace. After you have finished exercising, cool down for about 5 to 10 minutes. Again, stretch your muscles and let your heart rate slow down gradually. You can use the same stretches as in the warm-up period.

Walking

Walking is great. No expertise or equipment is required, you can do it any time and it's free! What's more, provided you do it regularly and for long enough, walking can be just as beneficial as any of the more vigorous activities (like jogging, etc.).

HOW TO START

- Take a 10-minute walk, twice a day.
- Gradually extend yourself.
- Walk every day.
- Walk for longer.
- Walk faster.
- Walk and swing your arms at the same time.
- Walk up one or two gentle slopes.
- Walk up steeper slopes.

Aim to walk briskly (swinging your arms) for 30 to 45 minutes, each day. This should include at least one reasonably steep slope. (*Please note*: This may take you several months to achieve, so don't be in a hurry.) Remember, exercise is for LIFE!

Swimming

For most people, especially those who are very overweight, swimming is even better than walking.

How to start and then extend yourself
As with walking, you should start by going to the pool twice a week for a gentle 15-minute swim. Gradually increase the length of your swim, and your work rate while in the water. Aim to build up to about 30 minutes a day, or 45 minutes twice a week.

Cycling/cycle-machine, or trampoline, or jogging

Your aim is the same as for walking or swimming. Start with a short easy routine – 10–15 minutes per day and gradually work up to about 30 minutes a day. Gradually increase your work rate, without ever straining yourself. If jogging, please invest in a good pair of running shoes that offer cushioned support, and if you're a woman, for all activities invest in a good sports bra.

If you haven't exercised for a while, it's really important to find a form of exercise you enjoy and to start slowly and build gradually. If you attempt 'too much, too soon' it will lead to soreness, fatigue and/or injuries. Work at your own level, start out slow, and gradually increase duration and level of difficulty as your body progresses.

In addition to your regular workouts, don't forget to do some gentle toning exercises as well – press-ups, sit-ups, lunges and so on. You need to be doing these for about 20 minutes three to four times a week. If you don't like going to a gym for a class there are plenty of fitness videos, books and magazines that can give you advice on how to perform toning exercises correctly. Failing that, try simple things like carrying your shopping more or walking up the stairs as these all help to tone your muscles. You could also try the exercises below that not only stretch and tone the muscles, but can help to relieve your IBS symptoms. (See also the yoga exercises in the previous chapter.)

Exercises

Abdominal training
Sit on the floor with your knees slightly bent and your back straight. You can hold your arms straight out in front of you for balance or you can cross them over your chest. From this sitting position, slowly roll back so that your shoulders are just a few inches above the floor. Pause and then slowly roll back up to a sitting position. As you do this exercise, always press the small of your back downwards, rather than arching your back, in order to prevent strain. Repeat ten times.

Stomach flapping
Stand up with your hands on your knees. Inhale and exhale fully. With your breath held out, pull your stomach in as far as you can, then release it all the way out. Repeat this flapping five times in one exhalation.

Abdominal windmill
Lie on your back. Bring your knees up to your chest. Place both knees to your right, touching the floor on your right side. Then, keeping your knees together, revolve to the left, touching the floor on your left side. If you need to hold your knees with your hands, do so. Repeat ten times.

Getting fit, like healthy eating, is not an overnight proposition, it's a lifestyle commitment. Sadly, only one-third of those who begin an exercise programme are typically still exercising by the end of their first year. The good news is that with some strategizing and planning, you can beat the drop-out odds and make a successful transition to a lifestyle that incorporates exercise. Here are some tips to help you stay motivated.

- *Find a fitness partner.* Studies show that exercise adherence is generally greater if the family or a friend is included in the commitment to exercise. Find a walking partner, play tennis with your spouse, or go rollerblading with the children.
- *Start an exercise log or journal.* An exercise log or journal is an excellent way to chart your progress and provide motivation. Nothing beats the feeling of success as you read through your accomplishments. Exercise logs can take on many forms: a calendar to record your workouts, a daily journal to record your feelings and goals, a computerized exercise log, or a log purchased at a book shop. The key is to select a log or journal that fits your needs and provides you with the kind of information that is meaningful to you.
- *Schedule your workouts.* Exercise must be a priority in order to establish it as a lifestyle practice. Make time for your workouts and schedule them on your daily calendar or planner.
- *Dress the part.* Wear comfortable clothes appropriate for exercising, they will help you feel like working out. If you exercise at a gym, put your exercise clothes in a bag and set it beside the door the night before. When it's time to head out of the door, all you have to do is grab your bag on the way out.
- *Entertain yourself.* If you exercise alone, consider using a portable music device to listen to your favourite music, or books on cassette, to help keep you entertained during your workout. Many pieces of exercise equipment have racks that fit on to the console to hold reading material. If you exercise at home, turn on some music or bring the television within viewing range.
- *Make exercise non-negotiable.* Think of exercise as something you do without question, like brushing your teeth or going to work. Taking the lifestyle perspective will help you make exercise a habit.

Massage

There are many types of massage, but all are thought to help improve circulation, calm muscle pain and spasm, and relieve stress. Some people with IBS find therapeutic abdominal massage to be extremely helpful.

Therapeutic abdominal massage for IBS

- Put a tablespoonful of massage oil to warm for ten minutes, e.g. on top of a radiator. Suitable massage oils are almond oil or grapeseed oil.
- Add one or two (no more) drops of one of the essential oils listed below.
- Lie down in a comfortable position and gently massage the oil into your abdomen using slow circular movements in a clockwise direction, i.e. up your right side, across your tummy button, and down your left side.
- Play some gentle music and relax while you massage. Nicer still, get your spouse, carer or friend to do it for you – very soothing!
- Oils for constipation – marjoram, rosemary, fennel.
- Oils for diarrhoea – chamomile, lavender, neroli.

(*Note*: Never use these oils neat; always dilute them in a massage/carrier oil (see above).)

Meditation

Research has shown that meditation can help to relax the body and many people with stress-related IBS find that it helps. There are numerous books, cassettes and classes that can teach you how to meditate, but even without formal meditation techniques it can help to take some time out of your day to sit or lie down and simply stop doing anything. To have a go at meditation yourself, find a quiet place where you won't be interrupted. Sit in a firm chair with your back straight and try one of the following forms of meditation, each with a different focus object.

Mantra meditation

For this meditation you choose a word such as 'peace' or a neutral symbol such as 'ommm' and repeat that word or sound each time you breathe out.

Gazing meditation

For this meditation you look at an object such as a flower or a book to keep your attention focused. Keeping your eyes relaxed, you then gaze, rather than stare, at the object. Don't think about the object, just look at it.

Breathing meditation

This involves focusing on the rise and fall of your breath. Draw a deep breath, focusing on the inhalation, pause before you exhale, then exhale and pause before you inhale again. Try to clear your mind of all thoughts except your breath.

Walking meditation

Focus the attention on each foot as it contacts the ground. When the mind wanders away from the feet or legs, or the feeling of the body walking, refocus your attention. To deepen your concentration, don't look around, but keep your gaze in front of you.

Before each session inhale deeply, and then exhale to release any tension. During your meditation, if thoughts about your daily life creep into your mind (which they will do), accept them and let them drift away. Try meditation for 5 minutes a day and then work up to 15 minutes a day; the more you practise, the better you will become and, hopefully, the more relaxed and calm.

Music therapy

Music is one of the most commonly used methods for stress reduction. A mind-soothing music definitely helps to relieve stress. Many studies have been done on the role of music in relieving stress, and it has been found that it is the rhythm or the beat of the music that relieves stress. While listening to music there is an increase in the depth of breathing, which provides more oxygen and therefore more energy to the body. Also there is a secretion of the neurotransmitter called serotonin in the brain which acts as a mood stabilizer. So what are you waiting for? Grab some soothing classical or modern music, put your feet up, and relax.

Reiki

The Japanese art of healing is based on a philosophy that the laying on of hands on different parts of the body can balance the mind and body and spirit by unblocking energy and helping the body to heal itself. Although no studies have shown Reiki to be of benefit to people with IBS, it's gentle and relaxing and some say it works wonders.

Relaxation

Performed correctly, relaxation exercises can lead to a profound feeling of calm. Simple ways to relax include sitting quietly with a book or a magazine for an hour while using an aromatherapy candle to fill the air with a relaxing aroma, chatting to friends, or having a candlelit warm bath with a few drops of relaxing aromatherapy oil. For a deep relaxation exercise like the one in the box below, which tenses and relaxes different muscle groups, you need to set aside half an hour, preferably after a long soak in a warm bath.

Deep relaxation exercise

Sit in a comfortable chair – reclining armchairs are ideal. A bed is OK too. Get as comfortable as possible – no tight clothes, no shoes, don't cross your legs. Take a deep breath; let it out slowly. Repeat this. What you will be doing in this exercise is alternately tensing and relaxing specific groups of muscles. After tension, a muscle will be more relaxed than prior to the tensing. Concentrate on the feel of the muscles, specifically the contrast between tension and relaxation. In time, you will recognize tension in any specific muscle and be able to reduce that tension.

Don't tense muscles other than the specific group at each step. Don't hold your breath, grit your teeth or squint! Breathe slowly and evenly and think only about the tension–relaxation contrast. Note that each step is really two steps – one cycle of tension–relaxation for each set of opposing muscles.

Do the entire sequence once a day if you can, until you feel you are able to control your muscle tensions. *Be careful:* If you have problems with pulled muscles, broken bones or any medical contraindication for physical activities, consult your doctor first.

1 *Hands.* The fists are tensed, then relaxed. The fingers are extended, then relaxed.

2 *Biceps and triceps.* The biceps are tensed (make a muscle – but shake your hands to ensure you are not tensing them into a fist), then relaxed (drop your arms down into the chair – really drop them). The triceps are tensed (try to bend your arms the wrong way), then relaxed (drop them).

3 *Shoulders.* Pull them back (careful with this one), then relax them. Push the shoulders forward (hunch), then relax.

---

4   *Neck (lateral)*. With the shoulders straight and relaxed, the head is turned slowly to the right, as far as you can; now relax. Turn your head to the left; now relax.

5   *Neck (forward)*. Dig your chin into your chest, then relax (straining the head back is not recommended – you could break your neck).

6   *Mouth*. The mouth is opened as far as possible, then relaxed. The lips are brought together or pursed as tightly as possible; now relax them.

7   *Tongue (extended and retracted)*. With your mouth open, extend the tongue as far as possible; now relax (let it sit in the bottom of your mouth). Bring it back in your throat as far as possible; now relax.

8   *Tongue (roof and floor)*. Dig your tongue into the roof of your mouth; now relax. Dig it into the bottom of your mouth; now relax.

9   *Eyes*. Open them as wide as possible (furrow your brow); relax. Close your eyes tightly (squint); now relax. Make sure you completely relax the eyes, forehead and nose after each of the tensings – this is actually quite tough.

10   *Breathing*. Take as deep a breath as possible – and then take in a little more; let it out and breathe normally for 15 seconds. Let all the breath in your lungs out – and then a little more; inhale and breathe normally for 15 seconds.

11   *Back*. With shoulders resting on the back of the chair, push your body forward so that your back is arched; now relax. Be very careful with this one, or don't do it at all.

12   *Buttocks*. Tense the buttocks tightly and raise your pelvis slightly off the chair; now relax. Dig your buttocks into the chair; now relax.

13   *Thighs*. Extend your legs and raise them about 6 feet off the floor or the foot rest – but don't tense the stomach; now relax. Dig your feet (heels) into the floor or foot rest; now relax.

14   *Stomach*. Pull in the stomach as far as possible; now relax completely. Push out the stomach or tense it as if you were preparing for a punch in the stomach; now relax.

15   *Calves and feet*. Point the toes (without raising the legs); now

relax. Point the feet up as far as possible (beware of cramp; if you get this or feel it coming on, shake your feet loose); now relax.

16 *Toes*. With legs relaxed, dig your toes into the floor; now relax. Bend the toes up as far as possible; now relax.

Now just relax for a while. As your days of practice progress, you may wish to skip the steps that do not appear to be a problem for you and, after you've become an expert on your tension areas (after a few weeks), you can concern yourself only with these. Relaxation exercises such as these will not eliminate tension, but when it arises you will know it immediately, and be able to 'tense–relax' it away or even simply wish it away.

Visualization

You can reduce stress with your imagination. Through visualization, which is basically putting your imagination to work, you simply ease stress by changing your thoughts. This technique builds on the idea that we are what we think; for example, if we think sad thoughts, we become sad, and if we think positive thoughts, we become more positive.

This is a simple visualization exercise that will enable you to relax deeply. It takes about 10 or 15 minutes. But once you've practised it a few times, you can call on it instantly whenever you're in a stressful situation, before things get out of control.

Sit in a chair. If it's comfortable for you to do so, keep your back straight. Breathe in through your nose to a count of four. Breathe out through your mouth to a count of eight. If you have some privacy, say 'huh, huh, huh' at the end of the exhalation. Repeat the breaths four times.

Close your eyes. Tighten the muscles in your feet and then relax. Concentrate on feeling the muscles relax. Repeat. Tighten the muscles in your calves, relax, feel the relaxation, and repeat. Do the same with the muscles in your thighs, then with your buttocks, stomach and lower back, then with your chest, then your upper back, then your shoulders, then arms, then hands, then neck. Make a face, scrunching up your facial muscles, relax, and then repeat.

Think of a peaceful setting. It can be a beach or a forest or anything. The important thing is that it is a place that you've been where you felt relaxed and happy and had an all-around 'good feeling'.

Remember what the place looked like. Picture the details in your mind. Then remember the sounds that you heard. Next, add in the smells. Then your sense of touch – what do you feel on your skin? Finally, add in the taste. Let all your senses work as you experience this place where you felt great.

Stay in this place in your mind for about five minutes, experiencing it as vividly as you can with all of your senses.

When you are ready, open your eyes. Stand up, lift your arms over your head and stretch. Drop your arms and shake them out.

At this point, think about the fact that you now know how to relax. It's a skill – a learned skill – and it is now in your repertoire of coping behaviours. The more you practise this exercise, the more skilful you will become. Then, the next time you're feeling angry or frustrated or upset, this is what you can do. First, be aware of what's going on with your body. Do you feel any muscle tension? If so where? Is your breathing different from the way it usually is? Is your heart beating faster? Do you feel any other changes in your body? Feel these physical symptoms that signal that you're under stress.

Stress is the body's natural response to danger. It floods the body with chemicals that prepare it to fight or to flee. This was very helpful in the ancient days when a danger might be something like a wild animal that you would need to fight or to run away from. But nowadays, many of the dangers that create stress are attacks not on our physical bodies, but on our sense of self-esteem. Neither fighting nor running are helpful with that, but still the body creates fight-or-flight chemicals, and now these chemicals interfere with your ability to cope. They can build up to such a great degree that they flood your system and keep you from thinking rationally.

So what you need to do, when you realize that you have the symptoms of being under stress, is to take a few deep breaths and recall the peaceful place that you experienced in the visualization exercise. Picture it again, vividly, in your mind. This will help your body cut down on the flow of stress chemicals before you become so flooded with them that you can't think straight.

Stress-busters you can use any time, anywhere

The following techniques can all help when stress threatens to trigger your symptoms and you haven't got time (or it isn't appropriate) to meditate, visualize for half an hour or go for a run.

Fill out your personal space

Shrinking away from other people creates tension, so consciously relax your body, starting with the shoulders, and letting yourself settle into your feet or your seat as if there were no one else around. Close your eyes or keep them slightly unfocused and turned downwards. Now imagine that you are expanding into the space just surrounding your body, flowing into it with every exhaling breath, taking more space for yourself.

Try the herbal remedy valerian

Valerian is a useful herb for stress-related anxiety and insomnia. This sedative has been shown to help people fall asleep faster, and to sleep better and longer without causing loss of concentration. Or drink some kombucha tea; this contains stress-busting B vitamins and other micro-nutrients and is made from a bacteria yeast culture.

Daydream

For five minutes every hour, try to 'shut down' and think of nothing but your perfect situation. This could be a dream holiday, ideal partner or simply thinking about doing nothing at all. You will be surprised at how effectively this can lower stress levels. Daydreaming is a natural stress-busting technique. Allow your mind to wander for five minutes if you feel tense – maybe using your favourite picture or happy memory to help you drift off.

Another type of visualization involves an image that you associate with tension which you can then replace with an image for relaxation. For example, you might visualize tension as a taut rope, the sound of thunder, the colour red, pitch darkness, persistent hammering, or blinding white light. These images of tension can soften and fade into images of relaxation. For instance, the taut rope loosens, the thunder subsides and is replaced by a light rain, red turns to orchid, the darkness begins to lighten, the pounding hammer is replaced by the murmur of cicadas and crickets, the blinding white light softens to a sunset.

Ayurvedic technique

Try this ayurvedic technique for soothing the brain: for as long as possible, gently massage the point above your nose in the middle of the forehead in a very light circular movement.

Aromatherapy

Certain aromas are thought to activate the production of the brain's feel-good chemical, serotonin. Drip a few drops of the following aromatherapy oils on to a tissue to sniff when you feel stress levels rising: jasmine, neroli, lavender, chamomile, ylang ylang, vetiver, clary sage. You may also want to use essential oils in your bath to help you unwind. When you feel tense, try one of the following: three drops of patchouli and three drops of sandalwood, three drops of rosewood and three drops of clary sage, or two drops of vetiver and jasmine. Or you might like to try two drops of peppermint or lemon essential oil on a tissue to inhale when stressed. If you prefer, you could also burn these oils in a vaporizer to help clarify and invigorate.

De-clutter

Mess creates confusion and a sense of loss of power. If your desk/home/car is messy and disorganized, have a good clear out and tidy up. You'll instantly feel more in control.

Release the tension

Do you hunch your shoulders when you are stressed? Do you tighten your fists? Do you cross your arms? Do you wrap one leg around the other? Become aware of the way your body reacts when you are under stress. Then when you feel yourself going into that stress position, do the opposite – release your shoulders, stretch out your hands, uncross your arms or legs, and don't forget to breathe. Stop frowning and relax your jaw by gently resting the tip of your tongue for a second behind your top front teeth. At the same time try to consciously relax the facial muscles and let the shoulders drop down and away from your ears by an inch or two – you'll be amazed to find how you were holding that tension in your body.

Chamomile

One of the best herbs for relieving tension is chamomile as it has a gentle sedative effect. Drink a cup any time you feel tense to help you to relax. If you drink a cup before you go to bed, this can help you to sleep.

Stroke your pet

If you have a pet, stroke it. It's been proven to lower blood pressure and stress levels. If you haven't got a pet, why not give someone you love a hug – it will have the same effect.

Write it down

When it all seems too much, grab a pen and paper and write down what you need to do. Listing things on paper will also help to focus your mind, helping you think clearly about what a priority is, what can wait, and what can be delegated to someone else. Once a job has been dealt with, be sure to cross it off the list. It's satisfying and stress-busting to watch your list shrink!

Get your head down!

Finally, one stress factor that can have a significant impact on IBS symptoms is sleep loss. Since a poor night's sleep results in fatigue and a corresponding lower stress-tolerance level, being tired allows IBS to be more easily triggered. A significant correlation has been noted between morning IBS symptoms and the quality of the previous night's sleep. In fact, morning IBS symptoms seemed to rise or fall in direct association with the prior night's quality of sleep. A less strong but still significant relationship was found between end-of-day IBS symptoms and the quality of sleep during the previous evening. Ensuring an adequate night's sleep should be a top priority for reducing stress-induced IBS symptoms.

So what is a good night's sleep? A good night's sleep boosts health and well-being, but research suggests that those who slept under six hours or over seven hours became irritable. Seven hours seems to be the most beneficial, but six hours of good-quality sleep is far better than a restless eight.

Everyone has different sleep needs, but if one or more of the items on the list below apply to you, you're not getting enough good-quality sleep:

- You yawn a lot.
- You fall asleep during the day.
- You lack energy.
- You feel drained or tired.
- You need caffeine and stimulants to get you through the day.
- You get dark circles under your eyes.
- You find waking up difficult.
- You find it hard to concentrate.
- You get irritable for no reason.

As well as eating healthily, there are many things you can do to improve your chances of a good night's sleep:

- *Keep regular hours.* Going to bed and getting up at roughly the same time every day will train your body to sleep better by getting it into a regular rhythm.
- *Keep a pen and paper by your bedside.* Use them to make a list before lights out of things that you need to tackle the next day, and thus 'dump' worries that may be preventing you sleeping during the night.
- *Get some fresh air.* Studies show that those who get their fair share of natural daylight tend to sleep better at night.
- *Take regular, moderate exercise.* Yoga, t'ai chi or simply going for a brisk walk or swim are all ideal. But note that taking vigorous exercise too close to your bedtime can hinder rather than help sleep.
- *Make sure that your bedroom is not too hot, cold, noisy or light.* An over-heated, under-ventilated bedroom can wake you in the middle of the night. Likewise, try to make your bedroom both as quiet and as dark as possible. A comfortable bed – not too hard, soft or small – and pillow will also help to create a good sleeping environment.
- *Avoid excess alcohol.* A small nightcap might help you to wind down and actually get to sleep, but alcohol is likely to interrupt your sleep later in the night.
- *Avoid coffee and tea – especially in the evening.* Both are stimulants, which can interfere with falling asleep and preventing deep sleep. Even the caffeine in fizzy drinks can harm sleep. Research shows that caffeine can also have an effect on some people if taken earlier in the day, so it may be worth looking at your overall intake, including morning and afternoon cuppas.
- *Avoid over-indulging.* Eating too much late at night can ruin your sleep patterns.
- *Don't smoke.* Yes, it's bad for sleep too. Nicotine is a stimulant, and smokers take longer to fall asleep, wake more often, and often experience more sleep disruption.
- *Drink a cup of herbal tea.* Unlike 'ordinary' (i.e. Indian) tea, this will relax rather than stimulate you.
- *Eat bananas and avocados.* Both are good sources of vitamin B, which can help with sleep problems that are caused by adrenal stress. You can also buy a good vitamin B complex – or astragalus, the herb favoured by Chinese healers – from a health shop and take it at bedtime.
- *Sprinkle a few drops of lavender oil on your pillow.* This is a natural soother.
- *Make love.* Sex is nature's best soporific. And, even if it doesn't send

you to sleep, it's a lot more fun than just staying awake and is also a fantastic tension reliever.

- *Try to relax before going to bed.* A warm bath – especially on cold, winter nights – will gently warm and relax you. A spot of yoga, deep breathing or listening to soothing music can also help to relax both the mind and body. Some people like listening to tapes of whale song or womb sounds. Your doctor might be able to suggest a helpful relaxation tape.

- *Use 'trigger pictures' to relax you.* Try to conjure mental images of a favourite or fantasy place or moment – such as, say, a great birthday party or an idyllic holiday spot – as a way of triggering feelings of relaxation and well-being.

- *Play mind games.* Counting sheep is the most famous such technique, but there are countless others, such as the following:

  - Imagine a room covered wall to wall and floor to ceiling with black velvet.
  - Describe your home village, town or city in the greatest possible detail, as though to a complete stranger.
  - Keep repeating 'Sleep, Sleep, Sleep, Sleep' very slowly until you drop off.
  - Numb the brain by making it perform a dull, boring task, such as repeating the words 'Um' and 'Ah' in ever increasing numbers. The 'Ums' must always be two more than the 'Ahs', giving the following sequence:
    1 Um
    2 Um Um Ah
    3 Um Um Um Um Ah Ah...and so on.

- *Don't just lie there, do something.* If you really can't sleep, don't just lie there fretting about it. Get up and do something that you find relaxing – reading, watching television or whatever – until you feel sleepy again. Then, when you start to feel tired, go back to bed.

8

Working with your doctor

Luke, 31
There's only one thing that relieves my diarrhoea and that is lomotil. I have to go to my doctor every few months for a fix, but it works. I don't like being so dependent on it, but I'd rather that than live my life running to the loo every half an hour. I hope I'll find another way one day, but my doctor thinks it's OK for me now.

Charlotte, 61
For about ten years I've had problems with constipation. I feel too young to have this problem and I was certainly too young when I got it. Doctors have constantly told me to include more fibre in my diet, but it hasn't helped and last year my doctor told me to take an antidepressant. I told my doctor that the reason I felt down was because I couldn't go to the loo like everyone else. He said antidepressant drugs might help, but they haven't. I've put on loads of weight and feel tired and thirsty all the time (typical symptoms of diabetes, though I'm told I don't have this). I don't feel like having sex at all. I thought being constipated was tough but this is much worse.

In many ways having IBS forces you to become your own doctor because it is up to you to take charge of your symptoms and find ways of dealing with them by watching your diet, taking more exercise and managing your stress levels. However, this isn't to say you don't need your doctor's advice. Far from it! Your doctor is the person you need to turn to for advice about managing your symptoms and monitoring any symptom changes that might need further testing. Teamwork between you and your doctor is essential, and a good relationship with your doctor provides an environment of understanding and concern that can make a huge difference.

Unfortunately, few doctors have specific training in how to manage IBS naturally with diet and lifestyle changes. Some may offer basic dietary advice, but for specific nutritional strategies and stress management techniques you'll need to read this book. Even so, your doctor is the person you should contact to monitor your symptoms and check your progress – especially if your symptoms change or you experience warning signs not associated with IBS, such as blood in your stools.

If your doctor does mention drugs as a treatment option, bear in mind that although drugs may be able to offer you short-term relief, they are rarely effective in the long term, because drugs treat the symptoms of IBS rather than the cause – that is, what is irritating the digestive system – and in some cases traditional treatments may actually make IBS worse. For example, drugs like Tagamet inhibit the release of hydrochloric acid in the stomach, but the change in stomach acid alters the microbial environment throughout the digestive tract and in this may actually exacerbate the digestive problems that caused the problems in the first place. Bear in mind too that drugs often have unwanted side-effects.

While the conventional approach to treating IBS has its downside, there may be times in your life when you need to resort to prescription medicine. So, listed below is a rundown of the most commonly prescribed drugs and what symptoms they are meant to treat, plus possible side-effects and concerns about them.

Over-the-counter medications for IBS

Many people with IBS, and doctors, turn to over-the-counter antidiarrhoea drugs such as Imodium, Maalox and Kaopectate for relief of IBS with diarrhoea. In a 2002 comprehensive report by the American College of Gastroenterology, researchers found these drugs to be effective in controlling diarrhoea. Such drugs, however, did not help with other IBS symptoms such as stomach aches or swelling. Side-effects of these treatments include stomach cramping, discomfort and enlargement, along with dry mouth, dizziness and constipation. If you take an anti-diarrhoea drug, use the lowest dose possible, and don't take it for an extended period of time.

Other over-the-counter products, such as Pepto-Bismol, antacids and medicines for wind relief, are considered safe. Tagamet, Pepcid and Zantac, taken for acid indigestion, are known as H2 receptor antagonists and their job is to prevent histamines from releasing certain chemicals into your stomach. By blocking this activity, stomach acid and acid indigestion is reduced. The problem is that stomach acids don't cause IBS, so popping these pills won't help in the long term.

Bulk-forming laxatives such as Citrucel, Konsyl, Metamucil and Serutan work by absorbing liquid in the intestines to help form a bulky stool that is soft enough to pass. These laxatives are generally considered a safe treatment for constipation, but can interfere with the absorption of some medicines. They can also stimulate some gas and bloating in the intestines.

Prescription medicines

Many of the following can only be prescribed by doctors, though some (e.g. Imodium) can also be bought over the counter.

Antidepressants

Doctors may prescribe antidepressants for the abdominal pain associated with IBS. This does not necessarily mean that you are depressed. Low doses of antidepressants are known to block signals of pain to the brain. For people with IBS diarrhoea, doctors will likely recommend a low dose of a type of antidepressant called tricyclic antidepressants, such as Pamelor, Elavil, and Tofranil. These drugs don't cause diarrhoea like some of the newer antidepressants, such as Celexa, Seroxat and Prozac. Common side-effects of these antidepressants include dry mouth, blurred vision and constipation.

It's important to note that the dosage of antidepressants used for IBS is typically far lower than that of the drug when used for depression. It is also crucial that the doctor prescribing this type of drug be very familiar with its use for IBS, as different classes of antidepressants have varying side-effects. Some can greatly worsen, instead of help, IBS symptoms such as diarrhoea, constipation and pain, depending on the individual. In particular, selective seratonin reuptake inhibiter (SSRI) antidepressants (Prozac, Celexa, Zoloft and Seroxat) stimulate serotonin production and can trigger severe IBS attacks in diarrhoea-predominant individuals, but they may be helpful for constipation. Conversely, tricyclic antidepressants (such as Elavil) have the best track record of success for reducing diarrhoea-predominant IBS symptoms, but those with constipation are usually not treated with these drugs because of the possibility of exacerbating this symptom. The long-term consequences of taking low-dose antidepressants for IBS are unknown, and this is a matter that should be discussed with your doctor.

Antispasmodics

Muscle spasms and gas in the gut cause much of the pain in IBS, and in some cases antispasmodics, like Donnatol, Levsin, Levbid, NuLev, Bentyl and Pro-Banthine, can help to relieve stomach cramping pain. Side-effects of antispasmodics include decreased sweating, constipation, and dryness of the mouth, nose, throat or skin.

Lotronex

Experts have found the prescription drug Lotronex (alosetron) to be effective for the treatment of all symptoms associated with IBS with diarrhoea, including stomach pain and distress, urgency and diarrhoea. The finding, however, was only relevant to women with IBS. Lotronex works to block the effect of serotonin on the digestive system.

Serotonin's role in the development of IBS is uncertain, but researchers do know that Lotronex somehow calms down the colon and slows down the frequency of bowel movements. However, in 2001 the FDA (Food and Drug Administration) took Lotronex off the market, due to its high risk of side-effects. As of March 2002, the FDA recorded at least 84 cases of ischaemic colitis, and 113 cases of serious complications of constipation (needing hospitalization) in connection with Lotronex. The severe side-effects resulted in four deaths. Yet Lotronex had gained strong support among doctors and patients who saw its value in treating the diarrhoea associated with IBS. Because of this, in June 2002, the FDA re-introduced the drug, but with several restrictions. Doctors now need to be enrolled in a special programme in order to prescribe Lotronex. The drug is approved only for women with severe diarrhoea-predominant IBS who have not responded to other treatments.

Imodium and Lomotil

These two drugs are the most common anti-diarrhoea medications for IBS. They enhance intestinal water absorption, strengthen anal sphincter tone, and decrease intestinal transit, thereby increasing stool consistency and reducing frequency. Both are meant to be used for the prevention of diarrhoea by taking them prior to events (meals or stress) that typically trigger symptoms. They should be taken with plenty of fresh water. Imodium can be used as a daily maintenance drug, but Lomotil is chemically related to narcotics, and as such is not an innocuous drug, so dosage recommendations should be strictly adhered to (especially in children). Lomotil can be habit-forming, and an overdose could be fatal.

Narcotic analgesics

Narcotic analgesics for IBS are opioid drugs and can be highly effective painkillers. One of their chief side-effects, constipation, is actually of benefit to some people with IBS. Narcotics also induce a feeling of tranquillity and promote drowsiness, both of which can be helpful for relieving stress-related attacks. The chief problem with narcotic drugs is that it's next to impossible to get a doctor to prescribe them for you. Although there is mounting evidence that these painkillers are not nearly as habit-forming as previously thought, from your doctor's point of view the risks of addiction are still likely to take precedence over your pain.

Zelnorm

This is a newly released drug just for IBS constipation in women, but it hasn't been on the market long enough to determine how effective (or safe) it is, and it's currently only supposed to be prescribed for short-term use. If you're considering taking this drug for IBS constipation, you'll probably find it helpful to get feedback from other Zelnorm users on the IBS Message Boards on the internet.

Calmactin (cilansetron)

This is a drug for diarrhoea-predominant IBS that is currently under-going clinical trials.

Visiting your doctor

When you visit your doctor you will want to know what is wrong, what the doctor can do to treat it, and what you can do to better manage it. He or she will begin by taking a history, asking for a description of the symptoms as well as possible factors that can bring them on or make them better. This will be probably be followed by a physical examination, possibly diagnostic tests, a diagnosis, and a discussion of treatment options.

Don't be afraid to ask questions; write them down before your appointment. As a person who has IBS, you should never feel devalued, ignored or uncomfortable with your doctor. If you do, or if your concerns are not being met, it may be time to change to another doctor. Your goal is to obtain a diagnosis, understand IBS and your symptoms, and to develop a management or treatment plan designed to meet your individual needs.

The course of IBS is highly individualized and can be challenging to even the most knowledgeable and caring doctor, so you need to be organized when you go to your doctor's appointment. Here are some things you can do to help make your visit to the doctor most effective:

- List your symptoms and how frequently they occur. Try to be as specific as you can. For example, describe where pain is located, how often it occurs, and what makes it worse or better. Keeping a daily diary for a couple of weeks that lists symptoms and associated activities can help to sort this out. Provide your doctor with a list of all other chronic illness currently affecting your health, or of prior infectious GI illness. List all prescription and non-prescription (over-the-counter) medications as well as herbal supplements you currently take. Include dosages and frequency.

- To avoid feeling flustered because of time constraints, jot down a few questions in a notepad before you have your appointment. Bring that notebook with you and use it to take down notes during the appointment. It is imperative that you walk away from your doctor's appointment with a clear understanding of what he or she tells you. Try not to be intimidated by your doctor and, if you have any concerns, such as a fear of cancer, talk about them immediately. In other words, do not be hesitant to ask questions. Make sure you understand what your doctor is saying and, if prescriptions drugs are suggested as an option, ask if there are alternative options. Don't ever feel pressurized into taking drugs.

Your best bet?

Your best bet is to find a doctor who understands IBS, and work together on monitoring and adapting your treatment plan, whether this involves prescription medication or not.

If you do decide to go down the drug route, bear in mind that no single drug is approved for all IBS symptoms, and their effectiveness can vary greatly from one person to the next. What particular drug will work best for you is something you and your doctor have to determine through trial and error. You should work in partnership with him or her to determine which medication best fits your needs. This might take a trial period of a few months and several follow-up visits or phone calls. If you do end up taking a drug and it doesn't work for you, don't feel that you are alone as many people diagnosed with IBS end up feeling more irritated than relieved after using them.

Many of those with IBS cite great frustration with the lack of safe, reliable and effective IBS medications on the market, and would like to see new options made available to them. Fortunately, there are currently numerous studies and trials underway, so keep your fingers crossed and your eyes open for new treatments on the horizon.

Finally, to help you with the doctor–patient relationship, look out for *How to Get the Best from Your Doctor*, by Dr Tom Smith (Sheldon Press 2007).

9

A to Z of specific symptoms and natural ways to beat them

Not everyone with IBS is the same. Eating healthily and working out which combination of diet and lifestyle changes recommended in the IBS Healing Plan suits you best will help to boost your health, but if you have specific symptoms this can be a special cause of concern for you. In this chapter you'll learn how to add in adjustments, supplements and power foods, either on their own or with natural therapies, to help you beat your particular symptoms naturally.

Safety first

It's always best to use herbs under the care of a healthcare practitioner who is familiar with herbal medicine and to inform your doctor about all supplements or herbal medicines you are taking. If you have a history of cardiovascular disease, diabetes or glaucoma, are pregnant (or are hoping to be) or are taking medication, use herbs and supplements only in consultation with your doctor.

The common symptoms of IBS discussed in this chapter are:

- Abdominal pain.
- Anxiety.
- Bloating.
- Constipation.
- Cyclical symptoms of IBS.
- Depression/low mood.
- Diarrhoea.
- Fatigue.
- Headaches.
- Heartburn.
- Nausea.
- Wind and gurgling stomach noises.

(If faecal incontinence is a symptom, see Chapter 10: Living with IBS.)

Abdominal pain

Pain is a defining feature of IBS. Most people can tolerate the diarrhoea and constipation, but when they also have to deal with gripping pain and spasms, they can't cope so easily. Pain from spasms can trigger diarrhoea and constipation. A build-up of wind can also cause pain as sensitive areas are stretched and twisted. Be guided by your doctor, but there are some things you can do to help ease the pain when it strikes, including:

- Place a hot water bottle or heated wheat bag on the abdomen.
- Soak in a warm bath. Take care not to scald yourself.
- Drink plenty of clear fluids such as water and reduce your intake of coffee, tea and alcohol as these can make the pain worse.
- Try over-the-counter antacids, to help reduce some types of pain.
- Take mild painkillers such as paracetamol. Please check the packet for the right dose. Avoid aspirin or anti-inflammatory drugs unless advised to take them by a doctor. These drugs can make some types of abdominal pain worse.

Regular exercise is one of the best ways to decrease your risk of abdominal pain. This is because exercise releases chemicals called endorphins that block pain signals from your brain. It's pretty difficult to get morphine, but you have a ready-made supply of endorphins waiting to be released. Far better to exercise than to find a dealer!

Certain types of chronic abdominal discomfort can in some cases be eased with pain management methods such as biofeedback, cognitive behavioural therapy, stress management, hypnosis, acupuncture or acupressure.

Healing herbs for abdominal pain include: ginger, aniseed, fennel, oregano, peppermint oil, chamomile and skullcap.

Essential oils of geranium, chamomile, lavender, melissa, neroli, petitgrain, peppermint, thyme, tea tree, ginger and cinnamon leaf are used traditionally as pain relievers for abdominal pain. Put 10–12 drops of any one of these essential oils in one ounce of a carrier oil such as olive or coconut. Shake well and then rub into the abdominal area.

(See also the sections on bloating, wind and heartburn in this chapter and the section on stress management in Chapter 6.)

Anxiety

Anxiety is a complex condition which has been described as a feeling of uneasiness in varying degrees. It is a condition with many facets and can be mild to extreme in intensity. Fear of an IBS attack can trigger anxiety, but just living life can be anxiety-producing for some people. In fact, anxiety can be a forerunner to depressive illnesses and should be treated as soon as practicable. In the early stages, the normal drugs prescribed by doctors for anxiety may be avoided by trying some of the following diet and lifestyle changes and herbal alternatives:

- Take time out for yourself when you find you are feeling anxious. Create your own special place where you can be alone, without responsibilities. Begin a journal and note your feelings.
- Swings in blood sugar can trigger panic and anxiety, so make sure you follow the IBS Healing Plan diet guidelines and eat little and often to keep your blood sugar levels and your mood stable.
- It is advisable to avoid tranquillizers, antidepressants, alcohol, cocaine and opium as these drugs may lead to dependence.
- Motherwort contains alkaloids, tannins and saponins that act as antispasmodics, and calm the heart and nerves without sedating.
- Passionflower is known to have sedative and analgesic properties, having a calming and restful effect on the central nervous system.
- Valerian root also affects the central nervous system, and has been used in Europe extensively as a sedative and calmative.
- Chamomile (German chamomile) is commonly and successfully used for anxiety and insomnia, in addition to easing indigestion and GI inflammations. Caraway is also helpful.
- Catnip and peppermint also have a sedative action on the nerves. Balm (*Melissa officinalis*) and common lavender (*Lavandula angustifolia*) are two more herbs that have been shown to be effective in reducing anxiety. Any good naturopath will be able to assist you with both the supply and recommended dosages of these herbs.
- Essential oils useful in the treatment of anxiety are: bergamot, chamomile, neroli, ylang ylang, melissa, frankincense, cedarwood, lavender, valerian, vetiver and rose.
- The slow movements and controlled postures of yoga improve muscle strength, flexibility, range of motion, balance, breathing, blood circulation, and promote mental focus, clarity and calmness. Stretching also reduces mental and physical stress, tension and anxiety, promotes good sleep, lowers blood pressure, and slows down your heart rate.
- Listening to your favourite music is a great method of reducing stress and relieving anxiety. Your individual preference in music will determine which type of soothing sounds will best reduce your tension and promote feelings of tranquillity. Pay attention to how

you feel when you hear a particular song or genre of music, and keep listening to the ones that produce a relaxing effect.

- Optimism can counteract the negative impact that stress, tension and anxiety has on your immune system and well-being. Often it is how you perceive things that determine if you get overwhelmed, both mentally and physically. Having a positive attitude, finding the good in what life throws your way, and looking at the bright side of things enhances your ability to effectively manage stress.
- Relaxing in a hot bath relieves sore muscles and joints, reduces stress and tension, and promotes a good night's sleep. Add some soothing music, soft lighting and naturally scented bath salts or bubble bath/ bath foam to create an inexpensive and convenient spa experience in the privacy of your own home.
- Relaxation techniques such as meditation and massage can promote tranquillity and ease anxiety and they might be worth trying out on a regular basis.

Anti-anxiety foods

Bananas. Women who are depressed or anxious tend to have lower levels of Vitamin B6, which is needed for the production of serotonin, which is the brain chemical that lifts mood. Low levels of Vitamin B12 and folic acid can also cause anxiety. To boost your B vitamins, eat plenty of oily fish, eggs, nuts, seeds, soya beans, bananas and leafy green vegetables.

Selenium-rich food. People who are deficient in the antioxidant mineral selenium also experience feelings of depression and anxiety. Selenium is found in lean meat, fish, shellfish, brazil nuts, grains (see advice on eating wholegrains in Chapter 4) and avocados.

Eggs. Zinc is essential for the body to convert tryptophan into serotonin, the feel-good chemical that can induce feelings of calm. Zinc is found in eggs and also in nuts, seeds, peanuts and sunflower seeds.

Oily fish. Not only does eating oily fish reduce your risk of getting Alzheimer's disease, but according to studies reported in 2003 by the US National Institute of Health, it reduces anxiety and depression as well.

Nuts and seeds. A handful of nuts and seeds eaten 30 minutes before a stressful situation can help lower anxiety levels by boosting the production of serotonin – that same feel-good chemical that we have mentioned a number of times.

Bloating

Over-the-counter remedies are not advised as they can leach valuable nutrients from your body, but if you do get fluid retention as an IBS symptom, there are a number of things you can do to help yourself:

- Cut down on your salt intake. Use less salt in your cooking, watch out for hidden salts in your foods, and look for other ways to enhance flavour – for example, by using herbs and spices instead.
- Increase your fluid intake. You need to drink more, not less, to help your body dilute the salt in your tissues and allow you to excrete more salt and fluid. Aim to drink at least 2 litres of water a day.
- Reduce the amount of caffeine in your diet. Caffeine is a diuretic, but it won't ease bloating because it hinders the secretion of excess salt and toxins from your body.
- Make sure that your diet includes sufficient B vitamins, especially Vitamin B6, found in bananas, lean meat, fish, nuts and seeds. This is a tried and tested remedy for water retention.
- Eat foods that naturally decrease fluid retention, such as asparagus, cider vinegar, alfalfa sprouts and dandelion flowers. And eat more potassium-rich food to bring down your body's sodium level (the two minerals balance each other out). Reach for those bananas, apricots, black beans, lentils, tomatoes, green leafy vegetables and fresh fruits. Keep your blood sugar levels in balance. When blood sugar levels drop, adrenaline is released to move sugar quickly from your cells into your blood. When the sugar leaves the cells, it is replaced by water and this contributes to that bloated feeling.
- Get moving. Moderate exercise will make you sweat and hasten the transport of water through your body.
- Studies at the University of Reading have shown the surprising effectiveness of Colladeen, a mix of grapeseed extract, bilberry and cranberry extract, for the relief of bloating.
- Dandelion and parsley are natural herbal diuretics packed with hormone-balancing nutrients that allow fluid to be released without losing nutrients.
- Aromatherapy oils can be helpful with bloating. Add fennel or chamomile to a warm bath and soak for 20 minutes for the best effect. You may also want to use juniper as a massage oil.
- Bloating is often caused by intestinal gas. Intestinal gas can result from eating gassy foods or swallowing air. Swallowing air while eating is often done unconsciously and may result in frequent belching during or after meals. To avoid swallowing air, slow down when eating, don't 'slurp' drinks, and don't talk while chewing. Also

try to avoid chewing gum, hard sweets, carbonated drinks such as soda pop, and drinking through straws.

(*Note*: If the abdomen is tender to the touch or hard, contact your doctor to make sure that there is not a more serious underlying cause for the bloating. Although uncommon, bloating can also be caused by ovarian cancer and ascites (the presence of excess fluid often associated with liver disease and also sometimes with cancer).)

Ways of beating foods that cause bloating

Olive oil. This promotes the overall absorption of nutrients while helping the digestive system to function more efficiently. It can help reduce bloating because it is very well tolerated by the stomach due to its high oleic acid content. The sphincter that separates the stomach from the oesophagus is less affected by olive oil than any other fat – which means less indigestion, less acidity and less bloating. Two tablespoonfuls of olive oil taken in the morning on an empty stomach also appear to have a positive effect on chronic constipation, another cause of bloating.

Soya yoghurt. Lactobacillus acidophilus is one of the friendly bacteria that live in the intestines. When eaten, it travels to the intestines and crowds out the harmful bacteria that may be causing symptoms of painful gas and bloating. One source of these bacteria is yoghurt that contains live, active culture. It's important to look for yoghurts that specifically say they contain live culture, as many types of yoghurts are heat-treated to kill the bacteria before being sold. For people who either can't tolerate dairy or who choose not to eat dairy, a number of very tasty soya-based yoghurts are currently available at many health food stores.

Fibre. Throughout the day, snack on other high-fibre foods like strawberries, blueberries, dried apricots and dried plums. But be careful that you don't add too much fibre too fast, or you'll feel even more bloated than before. Your body needs time to get used to processing the increased bulk.

Bananas. Bloating can also be relieved by Vitamin B6 which is a natural diuretic. Healthy foods that are rich in Vitamin B6 include bananas, alfalfa, lentils, oily fish, soya products, raw nuts and seeds, especially walnuts, green leafy vegetables, rye, turkey, oats and brown rice.

Fennel tea. You might also want to try the odd cup of fennel tea.

Just brew a tablespoonful or so of fennel in a tea strainer and drink several cups a day. Fennel tastes like liquorice and has anti-gas as well as antispasmodic properties, making it especially helpful for bloating. It's also a very safe herbal remedy that you can use daily without any risks.

Constipation

Nothing's moving, even though you know you have to move your bowels and may even feel as if you should empty your bowels. Everything in your body is sending you that signal. You feel bloated and have uncomfortable pressure, but when you try to go, nothing happens. Or, if you do finally go, it hurts.

It's not a good idea to use laxatives as the first line of attack when you're constipated. They can become habit-forming to the point that they damage your colon. Some laxatives inhibit the effectiveness of medications you're already taking, and there are laxatives that cause inflammation to the lining of the intestine. If you must take a laxative, find one that is psyllium- or fibre-based. Psyllium is a natural fibre that's much gentler on the system than ingredients in many of the other products available today.

Bump up your fibre intake by switching from refined foods to less-refined foods whenever possible. Switch from a highly processed cereal to a wholegrain cereal, move from heavily cooked vegetables to less-cooked vegetables, and choose wholegrain products over products made with white flour. Sometimes, a little extra dietary fibre is all you need to ensure regularity. Fibre is found naturally in fruits, vegetables, grains and beans (although refining and processing can significantly decrease their fibre content). To avoid getting wind, increase the fibre in your diet gradually, and be sure you drink plenty of water so the fibre can move smoothly through your digestive system. See also the advice on soluble and insoluble fibre in Chapter 4: Healing IBS with diet. Especially bear in mind linseed – try to take a teaspoonful in the morning and another in the evening; chew thoroughly or grind just before eating.

Here are some other dietary tips you may find helpful:

- *Blackstrap molasses.* Take 2 tablespoonfuls before going to bed to relieve constipation. Molasses is too high in calories to use it as a daily preventative, but on an occasional basis it can help to get you moving. It has a pretty strong taste, though, so you may want to add it to milk, fruit juice or, for an extra-powerful laxative punch, prune juice.

- *Walnuts.* Fresh from the shell, they may be just the laxative you need.
- *Beans.* Dried beans and legumes, whether they're pinto beans, red beans, lima beans, black beans, navy beans or garbanzo beans, are excellent sources of fibre. Many people don't like them because they can give you wind. Cooking beans properly, however, can ease this problem considerably. Soak them first, discard the soaking water, and then add ginger, cumin or fennel seeds to the cooking water. Make sure they're really soft before you eat them. Plus, if you add beans to your diet gradually, you'll minimize gassiness.
- *Oregon grape.* The root of this plant has been used safely since ancient times to overcome occasional constipation. Mix half a teaspoonful of Oregon grape tincture in water and sip slowly before eating for best results.
- *Fruit and vegetables.* Eat at least five servings of fruit and vegetables daily. Eat an apple an hour after a meal to prevent constipation. Apple juice and apple cider are also natural laxatives for some people. Bananas can ease constipation too. Try eating two ripe bananas between meals. Avoid green bananas because they're con-stipating, and try a handful of raisins an hour after a meal. Rhubarb is a natural laxative too.
- *Sesame seeds.* These provide roughage and bulk, and they soften the contents of the intestines, which makes elimination easier. Eat no more than ½ ounce daily, and drink lots of water with the seeds.
- *Garlic.* Eaten raw, garlic has a laxative effect for many. Eat it mixed with onion, raw or cooked, and with milk or yogurt for best results.
- *Hot water with lemon.* Drunk first thing in the morning, before you eat breakfast, may help to get things moving.
- *Honey.* This is a very mild laxative. Try taking 1 tablespoonful three times a day, either by itself or mixed into warm water.
- *Safflower, soya bean, or other vegetable oils.* These can be just the cure you need, as they have a lubricating action in the intestines. Take 2 to 3 tablespoonfuls a day, only until the problem has gone (i.e. not on an ongoing everyday basis). If you don't like taking oil straight from the spoon, mix the oil with herbs and lemon juice or vinegar to use as a salad dressing. The combination of the oil and the fibre from the salad ought to sort out your constipation.
- *Vinegar.* Mix 1 teaspoonful of cider vinegar and 1 teaspoonful of honey in a glass of water, and drink.

While your diet is most likely to be the primary change you need to make for constipation, there are some other lifestyle changes that can also help. Stress, lack of exercise, certain medications, artificial sweeteners, and a diet that's lacking fibre or fluids can each be the culprit. Exercise in particular boosts regularity as well. When you are active, so are your bowels – so the more sedentary you are, the more slowly your bowels will move. Here are some other tips:

- *Heed the call.* People sometimes suppress the urge to have a bowel movement because they are busy or have an erratic schedule, or because they don't want to use public loos. If at all possible, heed the call when you feel it.
- *Don't rush.* It takes time for your bowels to move, so allow sufficient of this and be patient. It *will* happen. If you do feel the urge but can't manage a bowel movement, avoid pushing and straining and perform the colonic massage technique listed below several times a day instead.

Colonic massage

Perform the massage either sitting on the loo or lying down with your knees bent. Make a fist with your right hand and massage your colon using a digging, circular motion with your knuckles. Start at the lower right quadrant of your abdomen (just inside your hip bone) and work up to under the right side of your ribcage, then straight across, then down the left quadrant of your abdomen. When you get to just inside your left hip bone, massage in towards your groin/pubic bone. The idea is to massage the length of your colon. This starts at the lower right quadrant of your abdomen and then up in a horseshoe shape under the ribs and down to the lower left quadrant of your abdomen. The rectal canal then extends from the lower left quadrant diagonally across to the groin (or pubic bone). Repeat this massage several times, experimenting with varying pressure and your massage technique. This is a fantastic technique that can be used by anyone during, or to encourage, a bowel movement. It also relieves colic in newborn babies by helping them to expel wind and stools.

Cyclical symptoms of IBS

Many women notice that their IBS symptoms worsen around the time of their period. This is because when a woman's period starts, levels of the hormones oestrogen and progesterone drop naturally and this shift can trigger diarrhoea, wind, bloating and pain.

Women with IBS have symptoms all month, but their symptoms can get worse the week before their period. This means these symptoms can get jumbled up with PMS symptoms of bloating, anxiety, food cravings, breast tenderness and mood swings, while their diarrhoea symptoms are worse during their period – mixed up with period pain and cramps. If you find that your symptoms get worse before or around your period, you can use that information to your advantage. For example, you can make plans based on the knowledge of your menstrual cycle – for example, you would probably not want to be stuck on an aeroplane in the middle of your worst week.

There are a number of natural ways to ease PMS and the most common ones are listed below. In general you will find that the steps recommended in the IBS Healing Plan to ease your symptoms will also help to ease any symptoms of PMS:

- *Change your diet.* Eat little and often, and choose foods that are rich in fibre. This will help to stabilize your blood sugar and to ease mood swings, anxiety, depression and fatigue. Reducing your intake of salt and caffeine can help to ease water retention and breast tenderness. Taking steps to avoid constipation can also help some women (see the advice on page 85), and you need to ensure you drink enough water (paradoxically, this too helps to ease fluid retention).
- *Try Agnus castus.* A number of studies have shown that this ancient herbal remedy will help to reduce both mental and physical symptoms in up to 90 per cent of women. Agnus castus works on the pituitary gland to regulate the production of hormones. Give it time, though, as it can take up to three months to work.
- *Take some gentle exercise.* Gentle exercise, like swimming or yoga, releases brain chemicals called endorphins that make us feel happy, more alert and less anxious. Try to exercise throughout the month, but exercising when PMS is at its worst should give you some immediate relief.
- *Take a dietary supplement.* Calcium and magnesium will balance your hormones and keep you calm. Vitamin B6 aids serotonin production. Several commercial PMS formulae contain all of these. Evening primrose oil is especially helpful for breast tenderness.

Depression/low mood

Everyone gets sad from time to time and having a chronic condition like IBS can wear down optimism and enthusiasm. If your mood is persistently low it is important to seek advice from your doctor to discover the underlying cause, but if it is IBS that is dragging you down, the following natural mood-boosters may help:

A 'positive voice'

In 2002 researchers from the University of Kent found that people's perception of their bowel disorder affects how they cope with the condition. If they think optimistically about their condition and their life they cope well, but if they think negatively the symptoms are often worse. If you analyse your thoughts you may be surprised at how negative they are. For example, if you drop something you might think, 'Gosh, I'm stupid.' If you bump into someone you might think, 'Why am I so clumsy', and so on. If you're struggling with your weight you might think, 'I'm fat and ugly.' Try to catch yourself every time you have a negative thought about yourself or the things you do – and counter the thought with one that is more positive, or realistic. If you drop something or make a mistake, try: 'OK I messed up, but what about all the times when I've got things right,' or 'I was looking where I was going, the other person wasn't', and if you feel very brave, go for, 'That wasn't my fault.'

List the positive

List all the good things in your life. They could be such things as a job you enjoy, a loyal friend, a fascinating hobby, your dog, the flowers in your garden, and so on. Now make a list of all the good things in yourself. Have a good think now as there is bound to be a lot more than you realized. You might be a good listener or a great poet or have a great sense of humour.

Find new challenges

Taking on a new challenge can be incredibly rewarding and can make you feel more positive about yourself. If you've always wanted to learn how to play the piano or keyboard, book some lessons. Consider taking up painting, singing, jewellery-making, writing – the list is endless. Or perhaps you might like to get some new qualifications or take up a course, or even a subject that is helpful with dealing with IBS – such as homeopathy, reflexology, massage and so on.

Physical activity

This can contribute to a sense of well-being. In fact, regular exercise is considered by some experts to be one of the most effective treatments for depression. Plan to do at least 30 minutes of gentle exercise a day.

Everyday boosters

Sing along to your favourite music, have a good cry to release excess stress, and have a good laugh. Laughter sends those chemicals called endorphins, which we've mentioned before, whizzing around your body to make you feel naturally high. So, do something to get you chuckling – anything from watching a funny film to phoning an old friend.

St John's Wort

This has been shown in numerous studies to demonstrate a significant improvement in depression, anxiety and insomnia. The herb is taken in daily doses of 2–4 grams, calculated to contain 0.2–1.0 milligrams of hypericin. Capsules containing 300 milligrams of the extract (and 0.3 per cent of the active ingredient hypericin) are typically taken three times a day. Consult your doctor if you are considering taking St John's Wort to be sure it is safe for *you* to take.

Ginger

Ginger has been a powerhouse in Traditional Chinese Medicine for thousands of years. It is a diaphoretic herb that decreases fatigue and weakness and is potentially valuable for depression. It is also helpful for digestion, and acts as an anti-inflammatory.

Bach flower remedies

Wild rose, larch, mustard, gorse and gentian help to alleviate feelings of apathy, resignation, despondency, inferiority, despair, hopelessness, discouragement, self-doubt and intense descending gloom.

Sunlight

This is vital for both physical and emotional health. Try to get 15 minutes of sunlight on your uncovered eyelids daily (remove glasses and take out your contact lenses) in the early morning or late afternoon. In the absence of sun, try sitting next to six to eight regular fluorescent tubes (2,500 lux) for 30 minutes each day upon waking.

Massage

Massage is often more effective than talk therapy for reaching and healing hidden traumas and relieving depression. Even a single session can have a dramatic effect.

Posture

Stand tall, smile with your whole face, and breathe deeply. You will either start to feel happier or make your rage/grief more visible and more easily accessed.

Sigh!

To energize yourself when depressed, you can sigh deeply many times; hold your arms out in front of you for several minutes; bounce up and down on the balls of your feet. Try it!

Foods that fight depression

Grapefruit. These are great for boosting liver function and easing depression. The more toxins your liver is exposed to, the more easily its detoxification systems are overloaded. If the liver is sluggish, excessive amounts of toxins find their way into the bloodstream and can affect the function of the brain, causing unpleasant and erratic mood changes, a general feeling of depression, 'foggy brain' and an impaired ability to concentrate or remember things.

Artichoke. This is liver protective and also has a bile-producing and bile-moving effect on the liver. When bile lingers in the liver, it irritates the tissue, creating inflammation and decreasing the ability of the liver to carry out its function so you are more likely to feel tired and depressed.

Watermelon. Studies indicate that red-pigmented, lycopene-rich foods – such as tomatoes, papaya and watermelon – improve liver health, and a healthy liver is essential for detoxification and physical, emotional and mental health and well-being.

Sunflower seeds. Minerals are essential for the growth and functioning of the brain. Selenium (high levels are found in seafood and seaweed) has been shown to improve mood significantly. Other sources of selenium include Brazil nuts, tuna and wholegrain cereals.

Oily fish/linseed. Fatty acids regulate memory and mood. The brain is made up of 60 per cent fatty acids. The omega-3 types (DHA and EPA) are essential to the optimum performance of your brain. Omegas are found in oily fish – for example, mackerel, tuna, herring, salmon and sardines, as well as other foods such as avocados, olives, raw nuts and seeds, and their cold-pressed oils. All these foods contain good mood stimulants and it has been discovered that levels of depression can be improved by introducing these healthy fats to your diet. Omega-3 types are also excellent intelligence- and memory-boosters. If you don't eat fish, try some hemp or linseeds instead.

Lentils. These are an excellent source of B vitamins and folate. Folate deficiency has been linked to an increased risk of depression, and a deficiency in B vitamins increases the risk of anxiety, insomnia and mood swings.

Water. The body deteriorates rapidly without water, and dehydration is a common cause of tiredness, poor concentration and reduced alertness. So ensure you get your recommended eight glasses a day!

Diarrhoea

If you suffer from diarrhoea, try to avoid taking any anti-diarrhoea medications until you have given the IBS Healing Plan recommendations, and the suggestions below, a chance to work. This is because acute diarrhoea is a common short-term problem that usually resolves on its own, and chronic long-term diarrhoea as a symptom of IBS responds well to dietary modifications.

Try some potassium-rich banana, apple sauce and dry toast until you feel better to help restore balance to your body. You can also use live yogurt to replace beneficial bacteria in your intestines. Here are some other suggestions:

- *Blueberries.* Blueberry root is a long-time folk remedy for diarrhoea. In Sweden, doctors prescribe a soup made with dried blueberries for tummy problems. Blueberries are rich in anthocyanosides, which have antioxidant and antibacterial properties, as well as tannins, which combat diarrhoea.
- *Chamomile tea.* Chamomile is good for treating intestinal inflammation, and it has antispasmodic properties as well. You can brew yourself a cup of chamomile tea from packaged teabags, or you can buy chamomile flowers and steep 1 teaspoonful of them and 1 teaspoonful of peppermint leaves in a cup of boiling water for 15 minutes. Drink three cups a day.
- *Potatoes.* This is another starchy food that can help to restore nutrients and comfort your stomach. However, eating French fries won't

help as fried foods tend to aggravate an aching tummy. Other root vegetables, such as carrots (cooked, of course), are also easy on an upset stomach, and they are loaded with nutrients.

- *Bananas.* Long known as a soother for tummy troubles, this potassium-rich fruit can restore nutrients and is easy to digest.
- *Orange peel.* Orange peel tea is a folk remedy that is believed to aid in digestion. Place a chopped orange peel (preferably from an organic orange, as peels otherwise may contain pesticides and dyes) into a pot and cover with 1 pint of boiling water. Let it stand until the water is cooled. You can sweeten it with sugar or honey.
- *L-Glutamine.* This is an amino acid and is another remedy for diarrhoea. For some people it works very quickly (within two to three days usually). It's virtually tasteless and dissolves easily in water. Start with ¼ teaspoonful per day mixed in cold or room-temperature water and drink it on an empty stomach. If that's not enough, increase to ¼ teaspoonful two or three times a day. Then increase the dosage gradually (if you need it) to ½ teaspoonful, then ¾ teaspoonful, up to 1 teaspoonful two or three times a day. L-Glutamine directly nourishes and heals the mucosal lining of the intestines and causes the bowel to reabsorb the water in your stools, thus reducing the number and frequency of bowel movements. Do not use if you have any liver or kidney disease.
- *Avoid diarrhoea-causing foods.* These include refined sugar, refined flour (white, bleached), hydrogenated fats, caffeine, and acidic, tomato-based foods like spaghetti sauce and pizza. Most people find coffee (regular or decaffeinated) highly irritating as well. Anyone with IBS should automatically avoid processed foods, luncheon meats or hot dogs, and foods with artificial flavours/colour, preservatives or MSG. Colonic massage is also an excellent way to reduce the frequency of bowel movements as the massage helps to move all the separate little stool deposits around the colon and out at once, rather than in many separate bowel movements (see the Colonic massage section above).
- *Keep hydrated.* You can lose a lot of liquid in diarrhoea, but you also lose electrolytes, which are the minerals such as sodium and potassium that are critical in the running of your body. So make sure you drink plenty of fluids. Whatever you choose to drink, keep it cool; it will be less irritating that way. Sip, don't guzzle; it will be easier on your insides if you take frequent sips of liquid instead of guzzling down a glass at a time.
- *Cut out caffeine.* Just as it stimulates your nervous system, caffeine

jump-starts your intestines. And that's the last thing you need when you have diarrhoea.
- *Say no to sweet treats.* High concentrations of sugar can increase diarrhoea. The sugar in fruit can do the same. Steer clear of greasy or high-fibre foods. These are harder for your gut to handle right now. It needs foods that are kinder and gentler. In short, stick as much as possible to the recommendations for diet in Chapter 4: Healing IBS with diet.

Although usually not harmful, diarrhoea can become dangerous or signal a more serious problem. You should see the doctor if:

- You have diarrhoea for more than three days.
- You have severe pain in the abdomen or rectum.
- You have a fever of 102 degrees Fahrenheit or higher.
- You see blood in your stools or have black, tarry stools.
- You have signs of dehydration.

If your child has diarrhoea, do not hesitate to call the doctor for advice. Diarrhoea can be dangerous in children if too much fluid is lost and not replaced quickly.

Fatigue

Tiredness or fatigue is often reported by people with IBS. All the natural therapies given in this book should help boost your energy levels, but the following suggestions may be particularly helpful:

- Make sure you balance out your carbohydrate load with some low-fat protein to avoid the sugar highs and lows that cause fatigue. In fact, balancing your blood sugar levels is the best way to fight fatigue and boost your energy levels.
- Step up your exercise routine as people who exercise regularly tend to feel more energized than those who do not.
- Eat foods that are high in fatigue-fighting potassium and magnesium. Prime sources include fruit and green leafy vegetables and nuts, seeds and beans. You also need to make sure you are getting enough iron-rich foods. Foods rich in iron include wheatgerm, dried fruit, shellfish, sardines, red and dark green fruits and vegetables. If you are a vegetarian, you may want to take kelp supplements.
- The B vitamins are crucial if you feel tired as one of the symptoms of a deficiency of the major B vitamins is lack of energy.
- Co-enzyme Q10, a substance present in all human tissue, is a vital

catalyst for energy production and if you are deficient in this you may feel tired. Food source of co-enzyme Q10 include: fish, organ meats (like liver, heart, or kidney), and the germ portion of whole-grains. You may also want to take 30 milligrams a day of co-enzyme over a period of three months.

• Ginger can boost energy levels. Use it fresh in your food as a quick pick-me-up. Cinnamon is another energy-boosting spice.

• Aromatherapy oils such as basil and rosemary can be helpful in mental and physical fatigue. Both are stimulating and renewing and you may want to add a few drops to your bath or use in a vaporizer in your room.

Refer to the recommendations for stress-busting and getting a good night's sleep in Chapter 7 as stress and lack of sleep can both cause fatigue.

If your fatigue persists, you may want to rule out hypertension, diabetes, candida, thyroid problems, anaemia and/or a food allergy. Consult your doctor.

Headaches

Missing meals or nutrients can trigger a headache whether you have IBS or not, so make sure you don't leave more than a few hours between meals and snacks.

See if you can find a pattern or a trigger to your headaches. When you get a headache, note what you ate, when you ate, and how you felt when you ate. Perhaps you are sensitive to certain foods. Watch out especially for foods such as cheese, red wine, chocolate, citrus juice or fruits that contain tyramine, phenylethylamine and histamine which can all trigger headaches. Unfortunately, symptoms often don't hit you immediately after eating these foods, so you need to keep a diary for several weeks to notice a pattern. Typical tension headache triggers include stress, fatigue, too much sleep, lack of exercise, and activities that require repetitive motion such as chewing gum or grinding teeth. Magnesium helps your muscles to relax and a defi-ciency can trigger headaches. So make sure your diet includes foods such as leafy green vegetables, nuts and seeds, dark chocolate and soya beans.

Also ensure your diet is rich in essential fatty acids – especially omega-3. Another study suggested that those with migraine showed a significant reduction in symptoms when they took omega-3 fish oils every day.

It's best to avoid over-the-counter painkillers as many of them contain caffeine. Also, you can develop an intolerance to them.

Learn to relax. By reducing muscle tension you may be able to ward off a fair number of headaches. Sit or lie down in a dark, quiet room for 20 minutes. Place an ice pack on your forehead. Tension headaches sometimes respond better to the application of heat. When headaches or migraines play a part in your life, try to regard them as evidence that the body needs time to be alone, to recharge. Lie in total silence, in complete darkness, and sleep, if possible, until the headache is gone. Regular exercise and stretching can prevent many tension headaches.

Treat yourself to a neck, shoulder and head massage. Whether it is a traditional massage or acupressure, releasing physical tension and improving circulation can promote feelings of well-being and even prevent headaches. Simply rubbing your temples can relieve pain.

Putting an ice pack on the area where the pain is focused can reduce the blood flow which in turn eases the pain. In some cases a warm bath can make those prone to headaches feel better, especially if an essential herb such as lavender is added. Other helpful oils include rosemary, which can stimulate blood supply to the head, and eucalyptus, which eases pain. Add a few drops to your bath or make up a massage oil to apply to a neck and shoulder massage.

Use a blend of relaxing aromatherapy oils as a massage oil or add a few drops in your bath. Lavender, chamomile and rosemary can all ease pain.

If you have a tension headache and can't get to a dark room to relax, put your hands around the back of your head and drop your chin on your chest. Press your chin down and hold for a minute. Then use your hands to turn your head to the right and hold for a minute. Then back to centre and hold for a minute, then to the left and then back to centre, again for a minute.

One study showed that 70 per cent of those who get migraines had less frequent attacks when taking the herb feverfew. The herb milk thistle may also be beneficial as milk thistle helps to improve liver function. Other useful herbs include cayenne, chamomile, elderflower, garden sage, ground ivy, Jamaican dogwood, lady's slipper, lavender, marjoram, peppermint, rosemary, rue, skullcap, tansy, thyme, valerian, wood betony and wormwood.

Don't ignore headaches that occur over and over again. They could be a sign of an underlying health problem. If you have tried various DIY measures or your headaches become more intense or persistent, ask your doctor for advice.

Heartburn

Heartburn is often reported in people with IBS. It is caused by burning stomach acid (generated by digestion) washing back up the throat and is best treated with a natural approach. To treat heartburn, you do not really have to spend a lot of money on anti-acid or reflux medication. There are many home remedies that are very effective in relieving discomforts brought about by heartburn.

One of the most common ways to treat heartburn is to dilute one tablespoonful of baking soda in a glass of water. For many years, baking soda has been recognized as one of the best solutions to heartburn. The good thing about baking soda is that it is cheap. If you use baking soda to treat heartburn, you will not need to spend a lot of money. Since baking soda is readily available in supermarkets, you do not need to go to see your doctor to get a prescription.

According to experts, apples are great acid neutralizers. For many years, people have used the natural antacids of apples to relieve the discomforts brought about by heartburn. The good thing about an apple is that you can eat as much as you like without getting any adverse effects. The more apples you eat, the better off you will be. Apples are very rich in fibre and vitamins that could help your body to remain healthy and strong.

You will need to discover your triggers. If you learn what brings on your heartburn, you can avoid the triggers and eliminate the condition. Avoid acidic foods and drink – for example, tomatoes, oranges, grapefruit, alcohol, lemons, etc. Also avoid chocolate, peppermint, spearmint, high-fat foods and caffeine – especially in the evening.

Avoid lying down or reclining for two hours after eating.

Gently massage your oesophageal valve by rubbing gently just under your solar plexus and stroking downwards towards your belly button.

When you go to sleep, lie on your left side. Your stomach opens up to your left and this encourages the food and acids to stay in your stomach and away from your oesophageal valve.

Herbs that can help to prevent heartburn include: black pepper, cardamom seed, coriander seed, fennel seed, peppermint leaf and liquorice root.

Nausea

If nausea is a common symptom, try some of the following natural remedies:

- *Lime juice.* For an immediate nausea stopper, mix 1 cup of water, 10 drops of lime juice, and ½ teaspoonful of sugar. Then add ¼ teaspoonful of baking soda and drink.
- *Onion.* Juice an onion to make 1 teaspoonful. Mix with 1 teaspoonful of grated ginger and take for nausea (so long as onion is not one of the foods that triggers your IBS).
- *Aniseed.* This helps to cure nausea and vomiting. Brew aniseed into a tea by putting ¼ teaspoonful in ½ cup of boiling water. Steep for five minutes. Strain and drink once a day. Or sprinkle some aniseed on mild vegetables such as carrots or pumpkin.
- *Cinnamon.* Steep ½ teaspoonful of cinnamon powder in 1 cup of boiling water, strain, and sip for nausea. Do not try this remedy if you're pregnant.
- *Cumin.* Steep a tea with 1 teaspoonful of cumin seeds and a pinch of nutmeg to soothe tummy troubles.
- *Fennel.* Crush 1 tablespoonful of seeds and steep for ten minutes in 1 cup of boiling water. Sweeten to taste with honey. Sip as necessary for nausea.
- *Ginger.* Without doubt, ginger is the best stomach-woe cure. Taken in any form, it can relieve nausea. Try ginger tea, gingerbread or gingersnaps.
- *Mint.* Mint tea relieves nausea. Simply steep about 1 tablespoonful of dry leaves in 1 pint of hot water for 30 minutes, then strain and drink. Don't toss out those mint leaves when you drink the tea. Instead, eat them. Eating boiled mint leaves can cure nausea, too.
- *Acupressure* has been found to be effective for reducing nausea. You can purchase in many pharmacies pressure bands to be worn around your wrists.
- *Chamomile.* If you get nausea along with digestive distress, try drinking chamomile tea three times a day.
- *Vitamin B6.* This can also help to quell nausea. Increase the amount in your diet, from foods such as spinach, tuna, banana and salmon, or take a supplement.

If, in addition to nausea, you are experiencing a loss of appetite and difficulty in swallowing, or pain on swallowing, you should contact your doctor immediately for advice.

Wind and gurgling stomach noises

Because burping and breaking wind is the body's way of getting rid of swallowed air, you can cut down on unwanted and potentially embarrassing burps by reducing how much air you swallow. Here are some suggestions:

- *Stifle it.* Sometimes, burping and breaking wind produce such an inordinate sense of relief that chronic burping will encourage the person to burp many times. It's better not to do this; repeated burping can trigger more burping.
- *Don't smoke.* Here is yet another reason to stop smoking. When you inhale smoke from cigarettes, cigars or pipes, you swallow excessive amounts of air.
- *Watch what you put in your mouth.* Chewing gum and sucking on hard sweets or lollipops stimulates air swallowing.
- *Mind your manners.* Avoid talking with your mouth full because this makes you swallow air, and the more air you swallow the more likely you are to burp or break wind.
- *Eat slowly.* People who gulp down food and drinks are swallowing excessive amounts of air. They're also crowding the stomach with too much to digest, which causes a gaseous build-up.
- *Relax.* Anxiety and stress can cause you to swallow more often, which increases the amount of air taken in. When you feel stressed, force yourself to breathe slowly and deeply.
- *Limit your drinking of fizzy drinks.* Drinking carbonated beverages, including beer, creates air in the stomach that has to come out, one way or the other.
- *Don't use straws.* Drinking through a straw increases the amount of air that you you swallow.
- *Stay active.* Don't lie down after you eat. Activity will force the burps and gas out instead of letting them build up.
- *Keep a diary.* Keep a diary, noting foods and beverages consumed, as well as specific incidents prior to the start of burping. You may discover that you are more burp- or wind-prone immediately after you eat certain foods, like dairy foods.
- *Ginger tea.* This can help relieve the need to burp or pass gas. Lemon juice may also help. The fruit papaya is full of an enzyme called papain that can get rid of whatever it is that is causing the gas. Peppermint and other herbs (carminatives) that soothe the digestive tract may also ease belching and decrease bloating after large meals.

If you are worried about the smell created by breaking wind, refer to the section on faecal incontinence in Chapter 10: Living with IBS.

Gurgling stomach noises

These can get quite loud and can cause social embarrassment. You may be able to laugh it off with friends, but it's another thing altogether when it happens during a critical business meeting. Doctors do have a word for stomach noises. It's called borborygmi, which basically means all the sounds that come from your digestive system as food, air and gas move through. If your stomach is trying to get your attention and you're tired of the turmoil, try these tips:

- *Sip some warm ginger ale.* Warm ginger ale may be just what the doctor ordered for a gurgling stomach – if the gurgles are caused by gas or air. Putting soda bubbles in your belly may help encourage gas trapped in your stomach to come up as a belch so that it's over and done with.
- *Sneak a snack.* Stomachs gurgle more when they are empty, so if you eat regular meals and snacks the problem can be avoided. You probably don't have time for a meal, but sneaking a snack should silence your stomach. If you're in a hurry, you could eat a cracker or a piece of bread. That could stop the noises from occurring.
- *Don't gulp.* Ever tried to take a deep breath to stop your stomach from gurgling? You may have made the situation worse. You're just taking in more air – part of the problem in the first place. So if you do take a deep breath or yawn, try not to swallow the air.

10

Living with IBS

IBS is a real challenge because it is such an unpredictable medical condition. You may wake up one morning and feel great, and then by lunchtime you are doubled up in agony and have an urgent need to go to the loo. It's no surprise then that some people with IBS become anxious about even leaving their homes. They may also be afraid to switch jobs, go to a restaurant, travel, or have almost any type of social life because they are worried that their symptoms might flare up when there is no loo in sight.

Louis, 38
It has been about eight or nine years since being diagnosed with IBS, and it has been nothing but hell for me. Going to work, I have to make sure that I know where a toilet is along the route, when going to the shops I go before I leave home, and then I sit in the car because I start to feel light-headed and as if I am going to be sick. Being at a party is the worst for me, because of all the people, and even at my own parties I feel ill. There have also been embarrassing times where I haven't been able to make it to the toilet in time, and for me, being over 30, it's not the nicest of feelings when you've soiled yourself. I'm still suffering with IBS, and would like to one day go into a shopping centre with my wife and do some shopping with her without having all these problems.

Hopefully, the information given in this book on diet, supplements, alternative therapies, stress management and working with your doctor will help you to feel more confident about your ability to take charge of your condition, become an active participant in your healthcare, and live your life to the full. However, for those days when you are scared to leave home in case you can't find a loo, or those mealtimes when you afraid of eating in case it triggers an attack, or those moments when you are worried about ever having a normal bowel movement again and being doomed to a life of misery, the aim of this chapter is to give you some extra tools and an extra boost of confidence to get you out of your home and on with your life. (For tips on eating in restaurants, refer back to Chapter 4: Healing IBS with diet.)

Faecal incontinence

If you've got faecal incontinence with your IBS – involuntarily breaking wind and losing some of your bowel contents at the same time – then this is probably one of your most feared events. This really isn't something you want to talk about with anyone because of the stigma attached. Working through the IBS Healing Plan will certainly help to ease this symptom, but if it's something you are prone to, then wearing a small panty liner, the kind women use on light days of their period, is a great confidence-booster whether you are a man or a woman. The panty liner has an adhesive strip that attaches to your underwear and there is absorbent material on one side and plastic on the other to prevent moisture from reaching your underwear. Panty liners are small, thin and easy to carry with you in a bag or even your pocket.

If your problem is bigger than the size of a panty liner, never resort to inserting a tampon into your anus or blocking the anus with a pack of tissues when you go out because these measures dry up secretions that your anus needs to stay healthy. Go for adult nappies or briefs instead – they come in various shapes and sizes for light or heavy incontinence. Many adult briefs are disposable and have absorbent material that neutralizes odours, as well as anti-leak cuffs. If you are embarrassed about buying them in shops, you can always say they are for an elderly relative or you can order them from the internet. OK, they may not look or feel that attractive, but if you want to get back to living your life to the full, you need to adapt. The chances are you won't even need them soon, and wearing them now is just your 'security blanket' so that you can stop worrying and get on with living.

(*Note*: As well as wearing panty liners or a pad, it also makes sense to carry in your bag some adult wet wipes and a change of underwear.)

Covering up odours

Embarrassed about leaving a bad smell behind, especially at work, in public loos, or in a friend's home? Remember you aren't alone; everyone has experienced this problem at one time or another. If you are concerned about lingering smells, make sure you flush several times and always carry in your bag a small can of air freshener, but don't use fruity-smelling odours as it just makes the smell worse. Try to buy a product that kills odours, not masks them. You could also try striking a match in the loo. This helps to mask the smell. (Do be careful and dispose of the spent match sensibly – dropping it down the loo may cause blocked drains and, remember, do not try this anywhere that a smoke detector has been fitted.)

Helping children and teenagers cope with IBS

Many of those with IBS first develop symptoms during their teenage years or even childhood years. Symptoms like stomach pain, diarrhoea, constipation and bloating are difficult for adults to live with, but if you also have to cope with peer pressure, new relationships, new schools, puberty and exams, it can make life very miserable indeed.

On top of this, teenagers often find that their parents, and even their doctors, do not take them seriously when they try to seek help. Tummy aches are mistaken for anxiety about school work or other problems. This is incredibly hard for the child as not only does he or she have the physical pain and discomfort to deal with, that child also has to get past the fact that everyone around them thinks they are 'faking it'.

Because of this problem, it is vital that parents pay attention when children or teenagers complain of problems 'down there'. Of course, most youngsters will try to get out of school once in a while, but very few will pretend to have embarrassing symptoms like diarrhoea or wind. In fact, it may have taken a great deal of courage for them even to admit to these symptoms in the first place. It's very important that when they do manage to talk about their problem, they receive a sympathetic ear.

If your child is complaining of stomach and bowel problems, it is vital that he or she receives a definite diagnosis of IBS from a doctor – bowel symptoms can mean IBS, but they can also mean a range of other disorders, so please get these ruled out before you assume that it's IBS. Once a diagnosis has been made, you need to help your child find some treatments that work for him or her. Many of the treatment approaches recommended in the IBS Healing Plan will apply to your children as well, but it is important to work alongside your doctor.

It is also especially important that you tell your child that he or she is not to blame for the symptoms and that IBS is not all in the mind. Having said that, stress and anxiety can be triggers for IBS, just as certain foods can be triggers for IBS, and so anything you can do to relieve stress may help to relieve symptoms to a certain extent. Remember that your child may be worried about not reaching a bathroom in time and having an accident, or having to leave class during schooltime and being made fun of. At all stages of your teenager's illness, the best thing that you can do is to support them and be there for them. If you are standing beside your child saying IBS is real and it is miserable but we are going to beat this together, then you should find that your child or teenager is much more hopeful and happy about the future and far more willing to work with you to find the best treatment option.

Travelling by plane, car or train

Travelling if you have IBS can be a frustrating experience. Even for healthy people, a trip takes planning, but travelling with a medical condition requires some special preparation for comfort. Don't be stuck at home because you're afraid to venture very far from a loo – learn how to travel without the stress.

Many public loos on motorways or trains aren't clean or well-stocked. Carry a little travel pack containing extra undergarments and trial sizes of toilet seat covers, wet wipes, antibacterial hand wash, extra toilet paper, and anything else you might need. If you need to make a dash, you can grab your little bag and be off!

If you think it will help you, and is feasible, pack a portable toilet. It may not be useful in urban areas, but when travelling off the beaten path it could be very helpful. When possible, arrange your meal schedule around your trip. If you know that you have to use the loo about an hour after a meal, be sure to leave enough time between your last meal and the start of the trip for that loo break. Ensure that your travelling companions know that when you say you need to stop and find a loo, you mean *now*.

Flying causes a great deal of anxiety for many people, but you can minimize this anxiety by booking your ticket several weeks or even months before your trip. When you book, ask for an aisle seat. If you're comfortable doing so, ask for an aisle seat close to the loo.

In your hand luggage pack extra undergarments, wet wipes, tissues and any other items you might need in an emergency, or in the event of a loo not being clean or well stocked. Also remember to pack a snack and some water – it's likely that you will not want to eat the food available in the airport or on the plane. Wear incontinence pants for an extra confidence boost.

If the airline did not give you an aisle seat, you can always politely ask another passenger to switch with you once everyone has boarded the plane. Some passengers who often won't mind switching seats include a person who is travelling alone, a group travelling together that has been separated, or another passenger who wants the window seat.

Sex

IBS is many things, but it is not the easiest condition to have, especially for women, when it comes to the question of sex. Intercourse may be painful even when you are not having an attack, and if you are having an attack, sex is the last thing on your mind. You may even be afraid to get into a reclining position if you suffer from diarrhoea, and if you have constipation, the last thing you want is someone on top of you.

The 'telling other people information' below may be helpful when it comes to talking to your partner about your condition. This is really important when your partner wants to have sex and you do too, but your stomach doesn't. Your partner needs to understand that your digestive system is sensitive and that your sudden loss of libido has nothing to do with them and everything to do with the fact that you need to rush to the loo. If your partner does not want to feel rejected/hurt, then he or she has to know about your condition, when to back off, and wait for a time that is more appropriate.

If your partner feels rejected because you seem to prefer the bathroom to him/her, then be sensitive to the hurt feelings involved and, when you feel better, think about initiating sex. Above all, do not use your IBS to avoid intimacy or make IBS replace the 'headache' excuse.

Painful intercourse

Many women with IBS complain of a painful 'crampy' feeling during sex. Because sex can be painful for many reasons, and several factors could be causing the experience of pain during sex apart from IBS, finding the solution can be a bit like solving a mystery (a very painful mystery).

First of all it might help to try to work out when the pain started, how long you have had it, and where and when during intercourse you feel it.

Explore on your own. Exploring sexual pain yourself is particularly good because you don't have to worry about a partner poking you the wrong way. You can be as gentle as you want to be, and you're always in control.

Use plenty of lubrication. One of the most common reasons for painful sex is lack of lubrication. There are all sorts of reasons why women experience vaginal dryness, menopause for example, but using a personal lubricant can be an easy and effective way to treat this problem and eliminate a major cause of painful sex.

Communicate with your partner. It can be difficult to talk about sex at the best of times, even for couples who have been together for many years. When it comes to talking about a difficult sexual issue, the communication can get even trickier. But communication is key to resolving painful sex. Even if the cause is entirely physical, and will go away with treatment, it's still important to talk with your partner about the pain you're experiencing and work out other ways for both of you to satisfy your sexual needs while you are being treated.

Experiment with different sexual positions. For some with IBS, pain during sex happens as a result of pressure on the abdomen. Try exploring different sexual positions and see if this alleviates some of the pain.

Consult your doctor or other healthcare provider. If you can, in most cases it is worth talking with your doctor about this. Even if the problem clears up (or seems to clear up), pain during sex can be a symptom of other issues, and knowing this can alert your doctor to other questions that he or she may want to ask.

Telling other people

Keeping your condition a secret from the people you care about and who care about you can lead to tensions and misunderstandings, which is just going to make your symptoms worse, so it really is important that you talk about IBS.

Telling a partner, new friend, or even an old one, about IBS is an embarrassing and personal subject that neither of you is likely to be comfortable with. But if you take time to think about with whom, why, when, how and where you will share your problems, it can bring you closer together.

Who? First of all decide if you really do need to tell this person. Every acquaintance and business associate does not need to know. You'll want to know a new friend for a time (at least a few months) before sharing something so personal. This person should be trustworthy and should be able to keep your condition in confidence if you ask them to.

Why? Think about the reasons your friend needs to know about your IBS. Is it because you need to share with someone or because you want to become intimate? Or perhaps you're spending a lot of time together, and they have noticed that you feel ill sometimes? Be honest with yourself about your reasons.

How, when and where? And once you do decide to tell your friend, make sure you talk in a quiet place where it's just the two of you without distractions or other people to interrupt. Start the conversation simply. Explain that you have health problems, and the condition is chronic (it will come and go). There may be times where you are unable to attend events or have as much energy as your other friends. But also explain that it does not mean that you don't want to spend time with your friends or have fun. You want to live as normally as you can. You may also want to express to your friend that you are not asking them to 'do' anything – except to be a good listener sometimes.

Only tell as much as you – and your friend – are comfortable with. You don't need to share every detail. If you're going to go on holiday with this person, they'll likely want to know about the 'loo problems', but if it's a friend from work, they might not want to know that you need to wear incontinence pants, etc.

There's no doubt it takes real courage to tell loved ones about your symptoms but, as Michael says below, the more people can talk without embarrassment, the easier it will become for others to talk about it.

Michael, 25

I still get embarrassed about my IBS, but I've crawled my way to a stage where I can mention it casually to my family and friends without any problems, and one day I hope to be able to say the word 'constipation' out loud without turning purple.

If everyone with IBS tries not to be embarrassed, we're not only making things better for ourselves, we're making things better for all those who follow us. Every time someone talks about their bowel movements in public, it enables someone else to do the same – and if they're talking about it, they're on the way to finding help.

And to the non-sufferers, I would ask you to consider your attitudes towards things like bathroom smells and flatulence. If your loved one has a terrible attack of diarrhoea and stinks up the bathroom – so what? You love this person, don't you? Is it their fault, or are they really suffering right now? If you take a matter-of-fact attitude to bodily functions, smells, noises and all the other nasty things we IBS-ers have to put up with, it will help your loved one realize that they are still loved, and will help you both recognize that IBS does not define a person – it's the way you live that counts.

At work, talking to a trusted supervisor or co-worker may make it easier for you to deal with the condition. Let them know that you have a valid chronic illness, and when symptoms flare up, you have no control over it. This might mean bringing in educational materials, or even this book, to explain about the condition. At the same time, tell this person that you've got a plan to deal with the syndrome (such as taking medication or going to the loo a few times), and that, despite it all, you'll remain a dedicated worker.

You may well find that once you do start telling people about your condition, most people are more supportive if you're upfront with them. In fact, more people today know about the syndrome and understand its implications than ever before, and media awareness is increasing.

There are other sources of support if you don't feel comfortable talking with people you know. There are doctors, nurses, therapists and dieticians who specialize in IBS and who can give you valuable feedback. You can also ask your doctor if he or she knows of any support groups. (The IBS Self Help and Support Group has meetings online at <www.ibsgroup.org.>)

Also, there are numerous websites for those with IBS. If you decide to log on and send an appeal or question to an online support group about something that worries you, you'll almost certainly get plenty of replies. Finding online support is easy. Just type the words 'IBS support group' into your search engines and you'll get dozens of websites coming up. Do be careful about buying products or following any medical advice from these websites, though, as they may not be medically approved or censored. If you do hear about a treatment that has worked wonders for someone, as Jo did below, make sure you check it out with your doctor first.

Jo, 37

I have suffered from IBS since I was about 15. I am now 37. At first I could cope with it as it was just occasional diarrhoea, but over the years it got worse and worse. I had all the usual tests done at the doctors, like everyone on this site has had, and I was eventually told it was IBS and I would have to live with it.

I tried many prescription medications to no avail, and also went down the alternative route, but again with no luck. It was ruining my life. I couldn't go anywhere without knowing there was a loo nearby. My friends, I know, used to get fed up with me as I was always running off to the loo on shopping outings or theatre trips. I have been caught short a number of times while out walking my dog (thank God for bushes!). I have even lost control in the kitchen of my house in front of my teenage son. I was absolutely mortified and cried and cried.

My saviour was an IBS support group on the internet. First, reading all about others with the condition and how much worse some are than me – and I thought I was bad enough – made me count my blessings a bit. Secondly, I heard about taking calcium for my IBS. I asked my doctor if it was worth a try and he said it certainly was, so I tried it and within two days this little (well big, actually) tablet completely changed my life. I no longer have diarrhoea, it has been three months now and not once have I had it. I go once a day now, usually in the mornings, and it is completely normal, a normal shape size and colour! I still can't believe it really, I feel like a normal person. I no longer get the spasms, the bloating, the sickness, no symptoms whatsoever.

If after reading this chapter you still feel nervous about leaving the house for long periods of time, having a social life or telling friends and loved ones about your symptoms, take things slowly at first. Invite people to your home, tell just one close friend, visit an IBS support group on the web, and go out of the house for short periods of time. The cinema might be a bit too long for an outing, but a ten-minute short walk around the park certainly isn't. When you start to discover that you can survive these shorter outings, you can start to feel more confidence about getting out of the house more and gradually increasing your time spent in public.

Run, don't walk

It is helpful at this point for you to remind yourself of the top ten things you need to do to manage your IBS. Tear out the page of this book (if it is yours, that is!) or write down these points and pin them on your fridge or loo door – anywhere that you will be able to read them often:

1 Every human being passes gas and has bowel movements.
2 Your bowel is normal – just irritable.
3 Your bowel needs routine to stay healthy, so eat regularly and get enough sleep.
4 Keep a food diary to identify food triggers.
5 Eat enough (but not too much) fibre (25 to 30 grams a day) and drink six to eight glasses of water a day.
6 Practise stress management techniques.
7 Get some fresh air and exercise every day.
8 One in five people have IBS; you are not alone.
9 Work with your doctor and talk about any concerns or fears you may have.
10 You can take control of your IBS symptoms.

Above all, pay attention to point 10: take control of your IBS symptoms so that they don't control you. This book has given you the tools you need to take control; it's up to you now to discover what works best with your IBS so you can start living again and running, rather than walking, towards your dreams.

Resources

If you suffer from IBS there are many resources that can offer you support, help and advice. In this section you'll find support groups, websites and books that can help you learn more about your condition and put you in touch with people who also have IBS.

UK

Core (the Digestive Disorders Foundation)
St Andrew's Place
London
NW1 4LB
Tel: 020 7486 0341
Website: www.corecharity.org.uk
Provides information and support for those with IBS and their families, and publishes a newsletter, leaflets and factsheets. If ordering by post, enclose s.a.e.

IBS Network
Unit 5, 53 Mowbray Street
Sheffield
S3 8EN
Helpline: 0114 272 3253 (6 p.m. to 8 p.m. Monday to Friday and 10 a.m. to 12 noon Saturday).
Website: www.ibsnetwork.org.uk
A UK national charity offering advice, information and support, including self-help groups. They publish a quarterly journal, *Gut Reaction*, which is free to members, and a 'Can't Wait' card to show in shops etc. when travelling or in an unknown town; this is available in a language of choice.

Australia

IBS Australia
PO Box 7092
Sippy Downs
Queensland 7092
Tel: 1300 651 131
Website: www.ibs-australia.org

Canada

The Canadian Society of Intestinal Research
855 West 12th Avenue
Vancouver
British Columbia V5Z 1M9
Tel: 604 875 4875
Website: www.badgut.com
Offers information, support groups and online support.

IBS Association
PO Box 94074
Toronto
Ontario MN4 3R1
Website: www.ibsassociation.ca
An organization dedicated to helping those with IBS via information, support groups, treatment and education.

USA

IBS Association
1440 Whalley Avenue 145
New Haven
CT 06515
Website: www.ibsassociation.org
A non-profit organization offering
support groups, information and
education.

IBS Self Help Group (IBS Group)
1440 Whalley Avenue 145
New Haven
CT 06515
Website: www.ibsgroup.org

**International Foundation for
Functional Gastrointestinal
Disorders (IFFGD)**
PO Box 170864
Milwaukee
WI 53217-8076
Tel: (414) 964 1799
Website: www.iffgd.org
A non-profit organization dedicated
to education and research.

Self-help websites

www.helpforibs.com
Help for IBS is a site owned by IBS
expert Heather Van Horous who
herself lives with the condition. It
provides information, education,
recipes and IBS-related products.
You can also sign up for online
support groups and message
boards.

www.ibstales.com
IBS Tales is a site for those with
irritable bowel syndrome to tell
their stories and read about the
experiences of others.

E-mail lists

If you join a mailing list server you
can receive e-mails from people
who are also dealing with IBS. Such
lists provide the opportunity to
communicate with others about
your condition. For example, the
following are both general lists that
are dedicated to IBS discussion:

health.groups.yahoo.com/group/
irritable-bowel-syndrome

www.health.groups.yahoo.com/
group/ibspag

Further reading

Braimbridge, S., and Jankovich, E., *Healthy Eating for IBS*. London, Kyle Cathie, 2005.

Brewer, S., and Berriedale-Johnson, M., *IBS Diet: Reduce Pain and Improve Digestion the Natural Way*. London, HarperCollins, 2004.

Burstall, D., *et al*. *IBS Relief: A Complete Approach to Managing Irritable Bowel Syndrome*. Hoboken, NJ, Wiley, 2006.

Nicol, R., *The Irritable Bowel Diet Book*. London, Sheldon Press, 1991.

Smith, Dr Tom, *Coping with Heartburn and Reflux*. London, Sheldon Press, 2006.

Van Vorous, H., *The First Year: IBS (Irritable Bowel Syndrome) – An Essential Guide for the Newly Diagnosed* (Patient-expert Guides). London, Constable and Robinson, 2004.

References

1 What is IBS?

Azpiroz, F. and Bouin, M., 'Mechanisms of hypersensitivity in IBS and functional disorders', *Neurogastroenterology Motility*, January 2007, 19(1 Suppl), pp. 62–88.

Kolfenbach, L., 'Pathophysiology, diagnosis, and treatment of IBS', *Journal of the American Academy of Physician Assistants*, January 2007, 20(1), pp.16–20.

Talley, N. J., 'Irritable bowel syndrome', *International Medicine Journal*, November 2006, 36(11), pp. 724–8.

2 What causes IBS?

Azpiroz, F. *et al.*, 'Nongastrointestinal disorders in the irritable bowel syndrome', *Digestion*, 2000, 62, pp. 66–72.

Bengston, M. B., 'Irritable bowel syndrome in twins: genes and environment', *Gut*, December 2006, 55(12), pp. 1754–9. Epub 2006.

Blumental, M. *et al.*, 'Herbal Medicine Expanded Commission E Monographs', *American Botanical Council with Integrative Medicine Communications*. First Edition. Newton, MA 2000.

Case, A. M. and Reid, R. L., 'Effects of the menstrual cycle on medical disorders', *Archives of Internal Medicine*, 1998, 158, pp. 1405–12. http://www.ama-assn.org/special/womh/library/readroom/arch98/ira70759.htm.

Eliakim, R. *et al.*, 'Progesterone and the gastrointestinal tract', *The Journal of Reproductive Medicine*, 2000, 45, 10, pp. 781–8.

Ewaschuk, J. B. *et al.*, 'The role of antibiotic and probiotic therapies in current and future management of inflammatory bowel disease', *Current Gastroenterology Reports*, December 2006, 8(6), pp. 486–98.

Fanigliulo, F., 'Role of gut microflora and probiotic effects in the irritable bowel syndrome', *Acta Biomedica*, August 2006, 77(2), pp. 85–9.

Garrigues, V. *et al.*, 'Change over time of bowel habit in irritable bowel syndrome: a prospective, observational, 1-year follow-up study (RITMO study)', *Aliment Pharmacology and Therapeutics*, February 2007, 1, 25(3), pp. 323–32. Epub 2007, 8 Jan.

Gilbody, J. S. *et al.*, 'Comparison of two different formulations of mebeverine hydrochloride in irritable bowel syndrome', *International Journal of Clinical Practice*, 2000, 54(7), pp. 461–4.

Jones, J. *et al.*, 'British Society of Gastroenterology guidelines for the management of irritable bowel syndrome', *Gut*, 2000 (Suppl II), 47, pp. 1–19.

Khosh, F., 'A Natural Approach to Irritable Bowel Syndrome', *Townsend Letter for Doctors and Patients*, 2000, 7, pp. 62–4.

Locke, G. R. *et al.*, 'Risk factors for irritable bowel syndrome: role of analgesics and food sensitivities', *American Journal of Gastroenterology*, 2000, 95(1), pp. 157–65.

Olesen, M. and Gudmund-Hoyer, E., 'Efficacy, safety, and tolerability of fructooli-gosaccharides in the treatment of irritable bowel syndrome', *American Journal of Clinical Nutrition*, 2000, 72, pp. 1570–5.

Oxol, D., 'Relationship between asthma and irritable bowel syndrome: role of food allergy', *Journal of Asthma*, December 2006, 43(10), pp. 773–5.

Playford, R. J. *et al.*, 'Bovine colostrum is a health food supplement which prevents NSAID induced gut damage', *Gut*, 1999, 44, pp. 653–8.

Quigley, E. M. *et al.*, 'Bacterial flora in irritable bowel syndrome: role in pathophysiology, implications for management', *Chinese Journal of Digestive Diseases*, 2007, 8(1), pp. 2–7.

Sanger, G. J., '5-Hydroxytryptamine and functional bowel disorders', *Neurogastroenterology Motility*, 1996, 8, pp. 319–31.

Shaheen, S. O. *et al.*, 'Frequent paracetamol use and asthma in adults', *Thorax*, 2000, 55, pp. 266–70.

Spiller, R. C., 'Role of infection in irritable bowel syndrome', *Journal of Gastroenterology*, January 2007, 42 Suppl, 17, pp. 41–7.

Tamboli, C. P. *et al.*, 'Dysbiosis in inflammatory bowel disease', *Gut*, January 2004, 53(1), pp. 1–4.

Varner, A. E., 'Reply to Locke et al.: risk factors for irritable bowel syndrome', *American Journal of Gastroenterology*, 2000, p. 3310.

3   Do I have IBS?

Chang, F. Y., 'Irritable bowel syndrome in the 21st century: perspectives from Asia or South-east Asia', *Journal of Gastroenterology and Hepatology*, January 2007, 22(1), pp. 4–12.

Garrigues, V. *et al.*, 'Change over time of bowel habit in irritable bowel syndrome: a prospective, observational, 1-year follow-up study (RITMO study)', *Alimentary Pharmacology and Therapeutics*, February 2007, 1, 25(3), pp. 323–32. Epub 2007, 8 Jan.

Kajander, K., 'Clinical studies on alleviating the symptoms of irritable bowel syndrome', *Asia Pacific Journal of Clinical Nutrition*, 2006, 15(4), pp. 576–80.

Kolfenbach, L. *et al.*, 'Pathophysiology, diagnosis, and treatment of IBS', *Journal of the American Academy of Physicians*, January 2007, 20(1), pp. 16–20.

Spinelli, A., 'Irritable bowel syndrome', *Clinical Drug Investigation*, 2007, 27(1), pp. 15–33.

4   Healing IBS with diet

Bijkerk, C. J. *et al.*, 'Systematic review: the role of different types of fibre in the treatment of irritable bowel syndrome', *Alimentary Pharmacology and Therapeutics*, February 2004, 1, 19(3), pp. 245–51. Review.

Bolin, T. D., 'Irritable bowel syndrome', *Australian Family Physician*, April 2005, 34(4), pp. 221–4.

Dapoigny, M. *et al.*, 'Role of alimentation in irritable bowel syndrome', *Digestion*, 2003, 67(4), pp. 225–33.

Drisko, J., 'Treating irritable bowel syndrome with a food elimination diet followed by food challenge and probiotics', *Journal of the American College of Nutrition*, December 2006, 25(6), pp. 514–22.

Farthing, M. J., 'Treatment options in irritable bowel syndrome', *Best Practice and Research Clinical Gastroenterology*, August 2004, 18(4), pp. 773–86.

Goldstein, R. *et al.*, 'Carbohydrate malabsorption and the effect of dietary restriction on symptoms of irritable bowel syndrome and functional bowel complaints', *Israel Medical Association Journal*, August 2000, 2(8), pp. 583–7.

Joung, Kim Y. and Ban, D. J., 'Prevalence of irritable bowel syndrome, influence of lifestyle factors and bowel habits in Korean college students', *International Journal Nursing Students*, March 2005, 42(3), pp. 247–54.

Kanazawa, M. and Fukudo, S., 'Effects of fasting therapy on irritable bowel syndrome', *International Journal of Behavioural Medicine*, 2006, 13(3), pp. 214–20.

Macdermott, R. P., 'Treatment of irritable bowel syndrome in outpatients with inflammatory bowel disease using a food and beverage intolerance, food and beverage avoidance diet', *Inflammatory Bowel Disorders*, January 2007, 13(1), pp. 91–6.

Watson, A. R. and Bowling, T. E., 'Irritable bowel syndrome: diagnosis and symptom management', *British Journal of Community Nursing*, March 2005, 10(3), pp. 118–22.

5 Healing IBS with supplements

Akobeng, A. K. *et al.*, 'Double-blind randomized controlled trial of glutamine-enriched polymeric diet in the treatment of active Crohn's disease', *Journal of Pediatric Gastroenterology and Nutrition*, January 2000, 30(1), pp. 78–84.

Aller, R. *et al.*, 'Dietary intake of a group of patients with irritable bowel syndrome; relation between dietary fiber and symptoms', *Anales de Medicina Interna*, December 2004, 21(12), pp. 577–80.

Aquino R. *et al.*, 'Plant metabolites. New compounds and anti-inflammatory activity of Uncaria tomentosa', *Journal of Natural Products*, 1981, 54(2), pp. 453–9.

Aquino, R. *et al.*, 'Plant metabolites. Structure and in vitro antiviral activity of quinovic acid glycosides from Uncaria tomentosa and Guettarda platypoda', *Journal of Natural Products*, 1989, 52(4), pp. 679–85.

Aquino, R. *et al.*, 'New polyhydroxylated triterpenes from Uncaria tomentosa', *Journal of Natural Products*, 1990, 53(3), pp. 559–64.

Arimi, S. M., 'Campylobacter infection in humans', *East African Medical Journal*, December 1989, 66(12), pp. 851–5.

Aziz, N. H., 'Comparative antibacterial and antifungal effects of some phenolic compounds', *Microbios*, January 1998, 93(374), pp. 43–54.

Beesley, A. *et al.*, 'Influence of peppermint oil on absorptive and secretory processes in rat small intestine', *Gut*, August 1996, 39(2), pp. 214–19.

Cavallo, G. *et al.*, 'Changes in the blood zinc in the irritable bowel syndrome: a preliminary study', *Minerva Dietol Gastroenterol*, April 1990, 36(2), pp. 77–81.

Chang, II. Y. *et al.*, 'Current gut-directed therapies for irritable bowel syndrome', *Current Treatment Options Gastroenterology*, July 2006, 9(4), pp. 314–23.

Chapman, N. D. *et al.*, 'A comparison of mebeverine with high-fibre dietary advice and mebeverine plus ispaghula in the treatment of irritable bowel syndrome: an open, prospectively randomised, parallel group study', *British Journal of Clinical Practice*, November 1990, 44(11), p. 461.

Fernandez-Banares, F. *et al.*, 'Randomized clinical trial of Plantago ovata seeds (dietary fiber) as compared with mesalamine in maintaining remission in ulcerative colitis',

Spanish Group for the Study of Crohn's Disease and Ulcerative Colitis (GETECCU), *American Journal of Gastroenterology*, February 1999, 94(2), pp. 427–33.

Fujita, T. and Sakurai, K., 'Efficacy of glutamine-enriched enteral nutrition in an experimental model of mucosal ulcerative colitis', *British Journal of Surgery*, 1995, 82, pp. 749–51.

Grigoleit, H., 'Pharmacology and preclinical pharmacokinetics of peppermint oil', *Phytomedicine*, August 2005, 12(8), pp. 612–16.

Hotz, J. *et al.*, 'Effectiveness of plantago seed husks in comparison with wheat bran on stool frequency and manifestations of irritable colon syndrome with constipation', *Medical Klin*, December 1994, 89(12), pp. 645–51.

Ionescu, G. *et al.*, 'Oral citrus seed extract', *Journal of Orthomolecular Medicine*, 1990, 5(3), pp. 72–4.

Jones, K., *Cat's Claw: Healing Vine of Peru*. Seattle, Sylvan Press, 1995, pp. 48–9.

Liu, J. H. *et al.*, 'Enteric-coated peppermint-oil capsules in the treatment of irritable bowel syndrome: a prospective, randomized trial', *Journal of Gastroenterology*, December 1997, 32(6), pp. 765–8.

MacMahon, M. *et al.*, 'Ispaghula husk in the treatment of hypercholesterolaemia: a double-blind controlled study', *Journal of Cardiovascular Risk*, June 1998, 5(3), pp. 167–72.

McKay, D. L. and Blumberg, J. B., 'A review of the bioactivity and potential health benefits of peppermint tea (Mentha piperita L.)', *Phytotherapy Research*, August 2006, 20(8), pp. 619–33.

Nash, P. *et al.*, 'Peppermint oil does not relieve the pain of irritable bowel syndrome', *British Journal of Clinical Practice*, July 1986, 40(7), pp. 292–3.

Nobaek, S. *et al.*, 'Alteration of intestinal microflora is associated with reduction in abdominal bloating and pain in patients with irritable bowel syndrome', *American Journal of Gastroenterology*, May 2000, 95(5), pp. 1231–8.

Pittler, M. H., 'Peppermint oil for irritable bowel syndrome: a critical review and metaanalysis', *American Journal of Gastroenterology*, July 1998, 93(7), pp. 1131–5.

Quigley, E. M. *et al.*, 'Probiotics and irritable bowel syndrome: a rationale for their use and an assessment of the evidence to date', *Neurogastroenterol Motility*, March 2007, 19(3), pp. 166–72.

Rees, W. D., 'Treating irritable bowel syndrome with peppermint oil', *British Medical Journal*, October 1979, 2(6194), pp. 835–6.

Sandoval-Chacon, M., 'Antiinflammatory actions of cat's claw: the role of NF-kappaB', *Aliment Pharmacology and Therapeutics*, December 1998, 12(12), pp. 1279–89.

Shulz, V. *et al.*, *Rational Phytotherapy: A Physician's Guide to Herbal Medicine*. New York, Springer-Verlag, 1996, pp. 187–90.

Simmen, U. *et al.*, 'Binding of STW 5 (Iberogast(R)) and its components to intestinal 5-HT, muscarinic M(3), and opioid receptors', *Phytomedicine*, 2006, 13 Suppl 1:51-5, Epub 2006, 14 September.

Tassou, C. C., 'Effect of phenolic compounds and oleuropein on the germination of Bacillus cereus T spores', *Biotechnology and Applied Biochemistry*, April 1991, 13(2), pp. 231–7.

Tomas-Ridocci, M. *et al.*, 'The efficacy of Plantago ovata as a regulator of intestinal transit. A double-blind study compared to placebo', *Rev Esp Enferm Dig*, July 1992, 82(1), pp. 17–22.

Torri, A. *et al.*, 'Management of irritable bowel syndrome', *Internal Medicine*, May 2004, 43(5), pp. 353–9.

Valberg, L. S. et al., 'Zinc absorption in inflammatory bowel disease', Digestive Diseases and Sciences, July 1986, 31(7), pp. 724–31.

Visioli, F. et al., 'Oleuropein, the bitter principle of olives, enhances nitric oxide production by mouse macrophages', Life Sciences, 1998, 62(6), pp. 541–6.

Walker, A. F. et al., 'Artichoke leaf extract reduces symptoms of irritable bowel syndrome in a post-marketing surveillance study', Phytotherapy Research, February 2001, 15(1), pp. 58–61.

Wong, P. W. et al., 'How to deal with chronic constipation. A stepwise method of establishing and treating the source of the problem', Postgraduate Medicine, November 1999, 106(6), pp. 199–200, 203–4, 207–10.

6 Healing IBS with complementary therapies

Bensoussan, A., 'Establishing evidence for Chinese medicine: a case example of irritable bowel syndrome', Zhonghua Yi Xue Za Zhi (Taipei), September 2001, 64(9), pp. 487–92.

Carmona-Sanchez, R. and Tostado-Fernandez, F. A., 'Prevalence of use of alternative and complementary medicine in patients with irritable bowel syndrome, functional dyspepsia and gastroesophageal reflux disease', Revista de Gastroenterología de México, October–December 2005, 70(4), pp. 393–8.

Chan, J. et al., 'The role of acupuncture in the treatment of irritable bowel syndrome: a pilot study', Hepatogastroenterology, 1997, 44, pp. 1328–30.

Fireman, Z. et al., 'Acupuncture treatment for irritable bowel syndrome. A double-blind controlled study', Digestion, 2001, 64, pp. 100–3.

Galovski, T. E. and Blanchard, E. B., 'The treatment of irritable bowel syndrome with hypnotherapy', Applied Psychophysiology and Biofeedback, 1998, 23, pp. 219–32.

Gholamrezaei, A. et al., 'Where does hypnotherapy stand in the management of irritable bowel syndrome?', Journal of Alternative and Complementary Medicine, July–August 2006, 12(6), pp. 517–27.

Harvey, R. F. et al., 'Individual and group hypnotherapy in treatment of refractory irritable bowel syndrome', Lancet, 1989, 1, pp. 424–5.

Houghton, L. A. et al., 'Symptomatology, quality of life and economic features of irritable bowel syndrome – the effect of hypnotherapy', Alimentary Pharmacology Therapeutics, 1996, 10, pp. 91–5.

Keefer, L. and Blanchard, E. B., 'A one year follow-up of relaxation response meditation as a treatment for irritable bowel syndrome', Behaviour Research Therapy, 2002, 40 (5), pp. 541–6.

Lim, B. et al., 'Acupuncture for treatment of irritable bowel syndrome', Cochrane Database Syst Rev, October 2006, 18(4).

Spanier, J. A. et al., 'A systematic review of alternative therapies in the irritable bowel syndrome', Archives of Internal Medicine, 2003, 163, pp. 265–74.

7 Healing IBS with stress management

Gupta, N., 'Effect of yoga based lifestyle intervention on state and trait anxiety', Indian Journal of Physiology and Pharmacology, January–March 2006, 50(1), pp. 41–7.

Keefer, L. and Blanchard, E. B., 'A one year follow-up of relaxation response meditation as a treatment for irritable bowel syndrome', Behaviour Research Therapy, 2002, 40(5), pp. 541–6.

Levy, R. L. *et al.*, 'The association of gastrointestinal symptoms with weight, diet, and exercise in weight-loss program participants', *Clinical Gastroenterology and Hepatology*, October 2005, 3(10), pp. 992–6.

Lustyk, M. K. *et al.*, 'Does a physically active lifestyle improve symptoms in women with irritable bowel syndrome?', *Gastroenterology Nursing*, May–June 2001, 24(3), pp. 129–37.

Orr, W. C., 'Gastrointestinal functioning during sleep: a new horizon in sleep medicine', *Sleep Medicine Reviews*, April 2001, 5(2), pp. 91–101.

Toner, B. B., 'Cognitive-behavioral treatment of irritable bowel syndrome', *CNS Spectrums*, November 2005, 10(11), pp. 883–90.

Villoria, A. *et al.*, 'Physical activity and intestinal gas clearance in patients with bloating', *American Journal of Gastroenterology*, November 2006, 101(11), pp. 2552–7. Epub 2006, 4 October.

Whitehead, W. E. *et al.*, 'Effects of stressful life events on bowel symptoms: subjects with irritable bowel syndrome compared with subjects without bowel dysfunction', *Gut*, June 1992, 33(6), pp. 825–30.

8   Working with your doctor

Chang, H. Y., 'Current gut-directed therapies for irritable bowel syndrome', *Current Treatment Options Gastroenterology*, July 2006, 9(4), pp. 314–23.

Dellon, E. S. *et al.*, 'Treatment of functional diarrhea', *Current Treatment Options Gastroenterology*, July 2006, 9(4), pp. 331–42.

Klein, K. B., 'Controlled treatment trials in the irritable bowel syndrome: a critique', *Gastroenterology*, 1988, 95, pp. 232–41.

Lacy, B. E., 'Irritable bowel syndrome: a syndrome in evolution', *Journal of Clinical Gastroenterology*, May–June 2005, 39(5 Suppl): S230-42.

Quartero, A. O. *et al.*, 'Bulking agents, antispasmodic and antidepressant medication for the treatment of irritable bowel syndrome', *Cochrane Database System Reviews*, April 2005, 18(2)

Tillisch, K., 'Diagnosis and treatment of irritable bowel syndrome: state of the art', *Current Gastroenterology Reports*, August 2005, 7(4), pp. 249–56.

9   A to Z of specific symptoms and natural ways to beat them

Carmona-Sanchez, R. *et al.*, 'Prevalence of use of alternative and complementary medicine in patients with irritable bowel syndrome, functional dyspepsia and gastroesophageal reflux disease', *Rev Gastroenterology Mexico*, October–December 2005, 70(4), pp. 393–8.

Cremonini, F. and Talley, N. J., 'Diagnostic and therapeutic strategies in the irritable bowel syndrome', *Minerva Medicine*, October 2004, 95(5), pp. 427–41.

Dellon, E. S and Ringel, Y., 'Treatment of Functional Diarrhea', *Current Treatment Options Gastroenterology*, July 2006, 9(4), pp. 331–42.

Fernandez-Banares, F., 'Nutritional care of the patient with constipation', *Best Practice and Research Clinical Gastroenterology*, 2006, 20(3), pp. 575–87.

Gerson, M. J. *et al.*, 'An international study of irritable bowel syndrome: family relationships and mind–body attributions', *Social Science and Medicine*, June 2006, 62(11), pp. 2838–47. Epub 2005, 7 December.

Kim, H. J. *et al.*, 'A randomized controlled trial of a probiotic combination VSL# 3 and placebo in irritable bowel syndrome with bloating', *Neurogastroenterology Motility*, October 2005, 17(5), pp. 687–96.

McKay, D. L. and Blumberg, J. B., 'A review of the bioactivity and potential health benefits of peppermint tea (Mentha piperita L.)', *Phytotherapy Research*, August 2006, 20(8), pp. 619–33.

Torii, A. and Toda, G., 'Management of irritable bowel syndrome', *Internal Medicine*, May 2004, 43(5), pp. 353–9.

10   Living with IBS

Amouretti, M. *et al.*, 'Impact of irritable bowel syndrome (IBS) on health-related quality of life (HRQOL)', *Gastroenterology Clinical Biol*, February 2006, 30(2), pp. 241–6.

Authors unknown, 'Is there any food I can eat? Living with inflammatory bowel disease and/or irritable bowel syndrome', *Clinical Nurse Specialist*, September–October 2006, 20(5), pp. 241–7.

Chiba, T. *et al.*, 'Quality of life in irritable bowel syndrome', *Nippon Rinsho*, August 2006, 64(8), pp. 1540–3.

Smith, G. D., 'Irritable bowel syndrome: Quality of life and nursing interventions', *British Journal of Nursing*, 23 November–13 December 2006, 15(21), pp. 1152–6.

Varni, J. W. *et al.*, 'Health-related quality of life in pediatric patients with irritable bowel syndrome: a comparative analysis', *Journal of Developmental and Behavioural Pediatrics*, December 2006, 27(6), pp. 451–8.

Index